Contents

PROCEDURES
in Skin Disorders

Lynette A. Stone
BA, RGN, RM(NSW), DMS
Clinical Nurse Manager—Dermatology
West Lambeth Health Authority
St. John's Hospital for Diseases of the Skin, London
& St. Thomas' Hospital, London

Eileen M. Lindfield
RGN, RM, OHNC, Cert. Dermatology,
Cert. Counselling
Occupational Heath Adviser, Camberwell
Heath Authority
Formerly Clinical Teacher,
St. John's Hospital for Diseases of the Skin
& St. Thomas' Hospital, London

Stuart J. Robertson
BA, ABIPP, ARPS, AIMBI
Director of Central Illustration Services,
U.M.D.S. of Guy's & St. Thomas' Hospitals
(St. Thomas' Campus & The Institute of
Dermatology), London

Wolfe Medical Publications Ltd

Copyright © L. Stone, E. Lindfield & S. Robertson, 1989
First published 1989 by Wolfe Medical Publications Ltd
Printed by W.S. Cowell Ltd., Ipswich, England
ISBN 0 7234 0912 9

A CIP catalogue record for this book is available from the British Library.

This book is one of the titles in the series of Wolfe Medical Atlases, a series
that brings together the world's largest systematic published collection of
diagnostic colour photographs.

For a full list of Atlases in the series, plus forthcoming titles and details of
our surgical, dental and veterinary Atlases, please write to Wolfe Medical
Publications Ltd, Brook House, 2-16 Torrington Place, London WC1E 7LT, England.

*H—indicates procedure should be used only in hospital, under medical supervision.

Acknowledgements

We would like to thank our patients and colleagues at St John's Hospital for Diseases of the Skin for their encouragement, support and co-operation; also Dr J.S. Dixon of Manchester University, for his permission to use Figure **1**, and the Institute of Dermatology, London.

Introduction

Most people experience various skin problems at some time. It may be a common ailment, e.g. a wart on the hand, a chronic disorder, e.g. psoriasis, or a rare debilitating genetic disease, e.g. dystrophic epidermolysis bullosa. Although the majority of people with skin conditions do not seek or need medical help, those who do may require specialist treatment.

Dermatological nursing is essentially an individualised process; patients respond differently to the same situations. In every case the nurse must be able to utilise all the specialist skills and techniques available in order to provide the highest possible standard of care. The role has four main facets:

— controlling skin conditions by carrying out prescribed treatments correctly;
— educating patients, their families or colleagues and the general public about skin disorders (prevention, control and treatment) and the promotion and maintenance of healthy skin;
— co-ordinating treatment between patient, skin care team and patient's family;
— providing psychological support to enable a patient to come to terms with his/her skin condition without feeling a social outcast.

We have included in this Atlas specialist practical nursing procedures used in the care of people with skin disorders. A few of them should be undertaken only in hospital and have been designated as such; all other procedures may be performed in hospital, consulting room or at home. A dermatological nurse can plan a total skin care programme with a patient who then should be able to continue to use the Atlas as a reference book when organising his/her own treatment.

1 Histology of normal skin

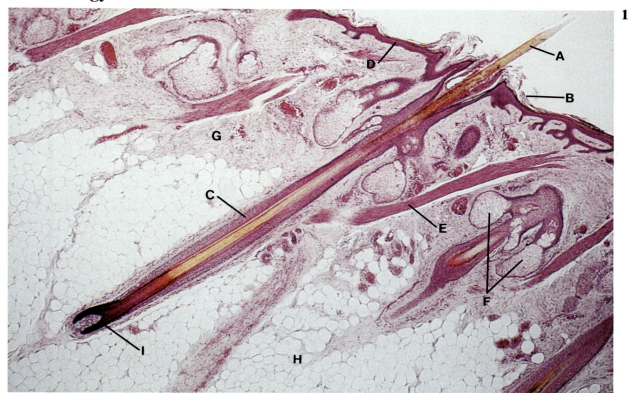

A	Hair shaft	**D**	Epidermis	**G**	Dermis
B	Horny layer	**E**	Arrector pili muscle	**H**	Subcutaneous tissue
C	Hair follicle	**F**	Sebaceous gland	**I**	Hair bulb

2a Terms used to describe skin change

Annular: Round or ring-shaped.

Atrophy: Wrinkled and silver white or reddened areas of sunken epidermis, e.g. discoid lupus erythematosus.

Bulla: A large elevated lesion containing fluid e.g. blister (Figure **74**).

Burrow: A linear lesion caused by parasites, e.g. scabies (Figure **138**).

Crust: Dead cells and serum, dried and situated over areas of epidermal loss or damage, e.g. impetigo crust (Figure **121**).

Discoid: Disc shaped.

Discrete: Separate lesions.

Erosion: Partial or total loss of the epidermis of the skin or mucous membrane, e.g. squamous cell carcinoma (Figure **2**).

Erythema: Reddened skin (Figure **51**).

Excoriation: Self-inflicted skin damage, e.g. persistent scratching caused by scabies infestation (Figure **139**).

Fissure: A split in the skin resulting from excessive drying or inflammation, e.g. split in skin with hand eczema (Figure **147**).

Generalised: Widespread eruption (Figure **36**).

Grouped: Clustered together.

Guttate: Drop-like.

Gyrate: Twisted spiral.

Keratosis: Horny thickening with defined edge (Figure **3**).

Keratotic: Horny thickening.

Lichenification: Bark-like thickening, accentuating the skin lines, e.g. in atopic eczema (Figure **77**).

Linear: Along a line.

Macule: A coloured spot, level with the surface of the skin, e.g. freckles.

Nodule: A large solid elevated lesion, e.g. nodular prurigo (Figure **4**).

Papule: A small solid elevated lesion, e.g. acne.

Pigmentation: Abnormal quantities of pigment in the skin— (*a*) hypopigmentation, e.g. vitiligo; (*b*) hyperpigmentation, e.g. post-inflammatory pigmentation.

Plaque: A well-defined elevated area, e.g. psoriatic plaque.

Polymorphic: Multiple types of lesions.

Pustule: An elevated lesion containing pus, e.g. pustular acne (Figure **10**).

Scale: Shiny, flaky and loosened skin on the surface of a lesion, or dry but otherwise unaffected skin, e.g. flaking skin in eczema (Figure **46**).

Scar: Any damage to the lower layer of the skin, the dermis, resulting in a scar formed from fibrous tissue, e.g. healed wound site.

Telangiectasia: Relatively permanent dilation of the skin surface capillaries (Figure **8**).

Tumour: A large solid lesion; it can be benign or malignant, e.g. seborrhoeic wart/basal cell carcinoma.

Ulcer: A lesion formed by local destruction of the epidermis and part or all of the underlying dermis, e.g. venous ulcer.

Universal: Majority of skin affected.

Vesicle: A small elevated lesion containing fluid, i.e. a very small blister.

Wheal: A solid elevated lesion formed by local superficial oedema, e.g. pressure urticaria (Figure **5**).

2

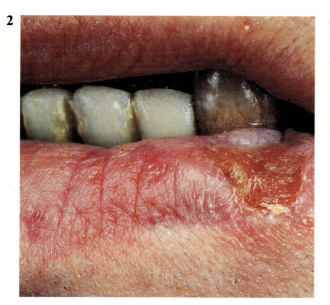

Erosion—squamous cellcarcinoma of the lip

3

Keratosis—solar keratosis

4

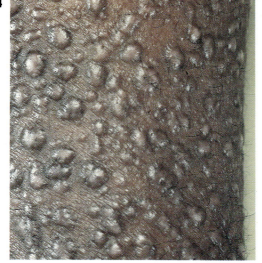
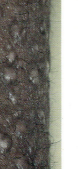

Nodule—nodular prurigo

5

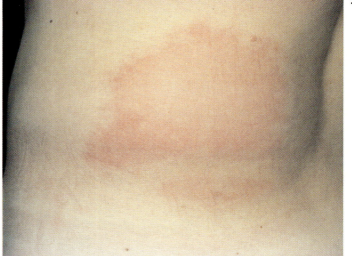

Wheal—urticaria

2b Recording skin state

Uses

To provide a framework of clearly understood terms.
To speed notetaking, reporting and assessment of progress during a patient's stay in hospital.

Equipment

Printed plan of method of lesion description.
Printed list of some common terms used to describe dermatological lesions.

Procedure

Outline method for describing skin state.

Areas involved	e.g. generalised (Figure **36**); localised (Figure **150**).
Type of lesion	e.g. primary (pustule); secondary or both (steroid exacerbated acne).
Formation	e.g. grouped; discoid.
Colour	e.g. erythematous (Figure **51**).
Unusual features	e.g. itching; pain; when the feature appeared; how long it lasted; how many times it has occurred; any aggravating factors involved; any burning sensation, etc.

3 Topical medications

Type of medication	Use	Note
Lotions Liquid vehicles for carrying medication; act by evapouration.	Cool through water evapouration. May be protective, anti-parasitic, anti-fungal, anti-pruritic; may act as sunscreen.	May be applied with cotton gauze or soft paint-brush.
Ointments and Creams Have greasy, non-greasy, or penetrating base depending upon nature of lesion and drug applied.	Lubricate. Protect the skin. Serve as vehicle for medications. Retard water loss. Used in chronic or localised skin conditions.	May have to be covered with a dressing to prevent soiling of clothing. Nurses should wear gloves when applying steroids to prevent absorption through the skin.
Powders (Usually with a talc, zinc oxide or cornstarch base)	Act as hygroscopic agents (take up moisture). Increase evaporation; absorb perspiration. Reduce friction.	Dispense with shaker top. Avoid accumulating powder in intertriginous areas.
Pastes Suspension of powder in a greasy base, usually soft paraffin.	Serve as a vehicle for medication, e.g. dithranol in Lassar's paste.	Remove old paste with liquid paraffin or vegetable oil. Apply thickly with a spatula to affected areas only. Dust with powder. Cover with tubular gauze.

4 Education of the in-patient

Uses

To reduce anxiety.
To teach the patient about his/her condition.
To enable the patient to participate actively in the treatment; assist staff and patient to solve any problems that may arise.
To ensure that staff can adapt the treatment to suit the patient's lifestyle and abilities.

Procedure

- Ensure privacy.
- Introduce yourself to the patient by name and smile. Do not hurry—allow time for patient participation.
- If space permits, sit at the patient's eye level while addressing him/her.
- Always speak in simple terms and avoid confusion caused by giving too many facts.
- Ensure skin contact with the patient during examination of the skin.
- Examine the total body area describing the amount, type and colour of lesions as specified page 20.
- From this initial information, assess the equipment needs and prepare the equipment accordingly—include all medications required, application instruments, dressings and protective coverings for furnishings.

- By the end of the planned programme, the patient should know
  — the name of his/her skin condition and its likely cause and course;
  — the type of treatment to be received during the stay in hospital and the effects and side effects of any medication to be given, e.g. tar may stain the skin and nails (Figure **6**).

Points to note

Use treatment time as a practical demonstration of treatment method.
Draw up a weekly or fortnightly programme introducing one new concept at a time.
Update progress records daily.
The assistance of another optimistic patient who has benefitted from similar treatment may be helpful.
The nurse should remember that many patients do not have manual skills, or possess knowledge of anatomy.

When the patient fully understands the procedure, it may be possible to commence teaching on self-administration of topical medication in preparation for discharge home. This is an individually paced activity depending upon the patient's motivation and ability.

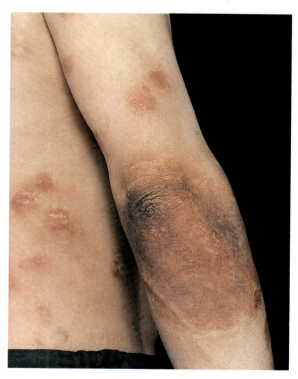

6

5 Preparation of a general skin treatment tray

Procedure
- Clean tray with cleaning solution.
- Line tray with paper to absorb any spillage.
- Place the following in the tray:
  Prescription sheet, covered with polythene.
  Small tray containing:
  > prescribed medication
  > gallipot
  > wooden spatula.
  Small tray containing measured and cut dressings.
  Two pairs of latex disposable gloves.
  Disposable plastic apron.
  Disposal bag.
  Scissors.

N.B. If treatment areas are allocated in the ward, a piece of paper will be required to cover the seats to prevent smudging of medications from patient to furniture. A piece of paper should also be placed on the floor for the patient to stand on.

---

6 General hints for ointment application

- Do not rub unless otherwise prescribed.
- Apply sparingly and never treat more frequently than prescribed; certain medications if over-used, can damage the skin, thus having the opposite of the intended effect.
- Apply in the direction of the hair fall as it lies on the skin (Figure **7**). This discourages folliculitis developing when ointment is trapped in the hair base. Ointments decanted into individual small pots help to prevent cross-infection.

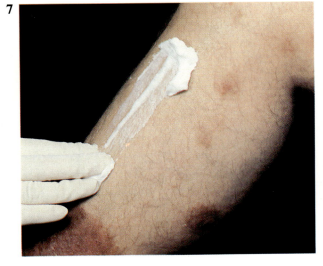

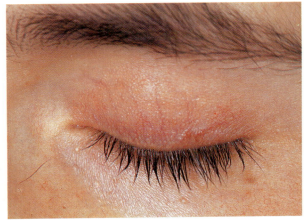

Topical corticosteroids

Use
To reduce redness of the skin surface by contracting the capillary vessels.

N.B. If used incorrectly potent topical steroids may cause:

- Thinning and fragility of the skin resulting in telangiectasia (Figure **8**);

- Redness of the skin due to permanent dilation of the surface blood vessels;

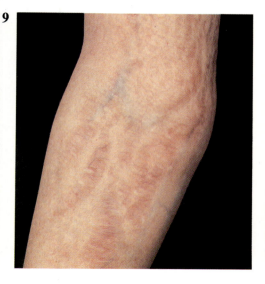

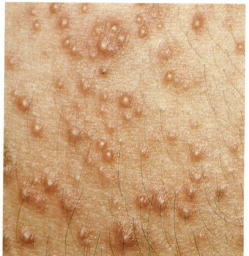

- Permanent stretch marks (striae) (Figure **9**);

- Delayed healing;

- Over-absorption of steroids via the skin, affecting the function of the adrenal glands;

- General masking of sensitisation reaction;

- Masking of fungal and bacterial infection;

- Exacerbation of pustular acne (Figure **10**).

- In order to prevent further damage to the skin, whatever the diagnosis, where practical try to avoid the use of adhesive tape to keep dressings or bandages in place. Never treat unaffected skin.

---

7 Sequence of medication application

A   Dithranol (Anthralin)
- Treat test area first (see page 32).
- Treat trunk; then apply tubular gauze.
- Treat upper limbs; then apply tubular gauze.
- Treat lower limbs; then apply tubular gauze.
- Change disposable gloves.
- Treat scalp.
- Change disposable gloves.
- Treat face, ears and neck.

This method avoids:

Unnecessary exposure of the patient.
Smudging the medication and burning the patient's normal skin.
Accidental burning of the nurse's skin.
Scales from the scalp adhering to an already treated face.
Facial cream being wiped off as the remaining dressings are being applied.

B   Creams and ointments
- Treat trunk.
- Treat upper limbs.
- Treat lower limbs.
- Apply tubular gauze to hands and arms.
- Apply tubular gauze to trunk.
- Treat soles of feet; then apply tubular gauze to feet and lower limbs. Ensure foot does not touch the floor between application of medication to the sole and application of tubular gauze.
- Change disposable gloves.
- Treat scalp.
- Change disposable gloves.
- Treat face and neck.

Any medication accidentally smudged should be wiped off immediately with vegetable oil, and the skin area washed clean.

8 Baths

Use
To provide overall cleansing and medicated treatment of a large area of the skin surface.

A Medicated types commonly prescribed

Type	Use	Quantity	Preparation	Note
Unguentum emulsificans (emulsifying ointment)	To cleanse and soothe tender skin.	As prescribed. Usual dilution 80cc to 120 litres of water.	Prescribed quantity mixed, then poured into bath water.	When left in a water-diluted state, can grow bacteria if exposed to air for a long period. As it creates a slippery bath surface, care should be taken when bathing.
Tar liquor picis carbonis	To aid in the preparation of skin for ultra-violet light exposure.	As prescribed. Usual dilution 60 ml to 120 litres of water.	Prescribed quantity mixed evenly in bath water with a gloved hand.	Stains nails, clothing and furniture brown. Use carefully as prescribed or directed. Tar may dry the skin.
Potassium permanganate solution in prescribed dilution	Anti-fungal antiseptic, drying agent for weeping or infected areas of skin.	As prescribed. Usual dilution 1:8000/ 60 ml to 120 litres.	Appropriate dilution is pink. Crystals should be fully dissolved before treatment. Mix in bath water with a gloved hand.	Can 'burn' inflamed skin if diluted incorrectly. Stains nails, skin, clothing and furniture brown or purple. Use as prescribed or for 3–4 days only.
Common salt	Cleansing agent for ulcers and infected skin lesions.	As prescribed. 1 kg to 120 litres of water.	Dissolve prescribed quantity evenly before treatment.	Can 'smart' sensitive skin. Do not wash hair or face in salty bath water.
Oatmeal	To reduce itching and soften skin.	As prescribed. 1 packet of prepared product; or 1 cupful or raw oatmeal.	Dissolve packet contents evenly in bath water; or use fresh oatmeal in a clear muslin bag as soap.	Fresh oatmeal grains are replaced for each bath.

B Assisted bathing

Procedure
- Check that the temperature of the bathroom is approximately 75°-80°F (24°-26°C).
- Check that all doors and windows are closed and no draughts exist.
- Check that the bath is clean and a fresh paper bath mat is put out.
- Accompany patient to the bathroom. Run bath (approx. 97°F/36°C). IT IS ESSENTIAL TO STIR IN THE PRESCRIBED AMOUNT OF MEDICATION AND MIX WELL TO ENSURE AN EVEN CONCENTRATION. Assist with removal of dressings and help patient into bath.
- Wash only below the patient's neck line.
- Leave patient to soak for 10 minutes. Pull bath plug out. Assist patient out of bath.
- Dry skin thoroughly, dabbing with a fresh towel.
- Dressings are sometimes applied in the bathroom to prevent rubbing of the skin surface against clothing.
- Accompany the dressed patient back to bed to rest.

Advice to nurse/patient

In-patient treatment

Always report any discomfort to the nurse or doctor.
Bath treatments may be changed regularly by the doctor according to the state of the skin.
Disposable plastic bath-liners may be used to reduce the risk of cross-infection and staining of the bath (Figure **11**).
The bath may be slippery, particularly when emollients are added to the water. Care should be taken when getting in or out of the bath. Where possible non-slip bath mats should be used.
When plastic bath-liners are used, care should be taken with children and sedated patients to avoid suffocation.
The face and hair are never washed in medicated bath water; they are always washed separately.

Out-patient/home care treatment

Do not continue with a bath treatment which you feel is unsuited to your skin. Return to the doctor and discuss.
Medicated baths usually last for a limited period only, unless bland substances, e.g. emollients, are used.
Never wash the face or hair in the same water that you have bathed in, as the previous day's skin medication has been washed off in the bath water. Clean water should be used for washing face and hair.
Never take a bath without assistance if taking medicine that causes drowsiness.
Do not allow children to bath without assistance in a medicated bath.
Care must be taken to avoid splashing bath water in the eyes. If accidental splashes occur, wash the eyes under cold running water for 15–20 minutes and seek medical aid immediately.

C Emollient baths

Use
To lubricate the skin and help to reduce irritation in dry and eczematous conditions.

Equipment
2 dessertspoonfuls of emollient (e.g. emulsifying ointment, aqueous cream).
Jug of boiling water.
Fork or whisk.
Half-filled tub—water should be at a comfortable temperature (approx. 97^0F/36^0C).

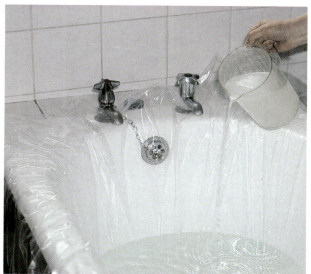

Procedure
- Explain the procedure to the patient.
- Dissolve emollient in boiling water. Whisk with a fork until it is completely dissolved. Add to the warm bath water and mix well.
- Warn patient to take care as the bath may be slippery.
- Patient should soak in the bath for 10 minutes.
- After bath gently *pat* skin dry. DO NOT RUB.

Advice to patient
Keep the bathroom warm as temperature changes may aggravate the skin.
Do not melt the emollient in a saucepan.
Use a bath mat to avoid slipping.
Wear light loose clothing after the bath.

Medicated soaks
These medications may also be used as indicated in the table above to treat small affected areas eg. potassium permanganate soak for hands or feet.

A plastic bucket or bowl lined with a disposable plastic bin-liner may be used. This
provides a conveniently sized container
avoids cross-infection
avoids staining the container.

9   Scalp treatment

Use
To treat scalp and hair conditions.

Equipment
Paper-lined tray containing:
Prescribed medication in tray.
Prescription sheet covered with polythene.
Disposable plastic apron.
Disposable latex gloves.
Disposable gallipot.
Clean comb.
Paper to cover shoulders.

Procedure
- Explain the procedure to the patient.
- Fix paper shoulder cover in place to stop scales falling on to the already treated skin of the body and limbs.
- Decant required amount of prescribed medication into a gallipot.
- Apply medication with gloved hand, taking a small quantity from the gallipot at a time.
- Divide hair into small combed sections and methodically treat all the affected areas (Figure **12**).

Advice to nurse/patient
Treat the scalp before the face as this reduces the amount of scales falling from the scalp and settling on the face.
Hair should always be washed daily while receiving scalp treatment unless otherwise prescribed.
When washing the scalp, use latex gloves to prevent unnecessary exposure to medication. It is preferable to use a shower attachment to the tap.
Care must be taken to ensure that the scalp is well exposed to the medication which is for scalp treatment and not usually hair treatment.

12

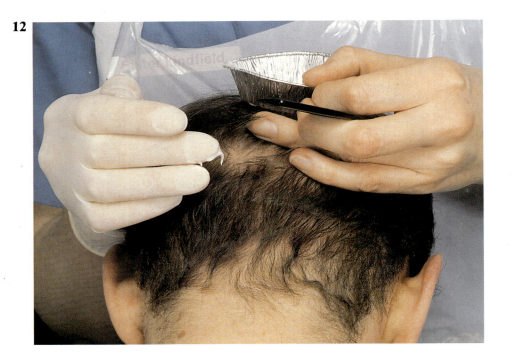

10   Shampoo treatment

Use
To clean hair and/or apply medication to the hair and scalp, e.g. in psoriasis of the scalp (Figure 13).

Equipment
Clean brush and comb.
Prescribed shampoo.
Plastic cape.
Towel.

Procedure
- Explain the procedure to the patient and seat him/her in a comfortable position.
- Place cape and towel around the patient's shoulders to protect clothing.
- Wet the hair thoroughly with warm water.
- Massage up to 10ml shampoo into the wet hair and scalp.
- If a medicated shampoo is being applied it should be left on the scalp for the prescribed time (usually at least 4 minutes).
- Rinse the head thoroughly with warm tap water to remove the shampoo.
- Massage a second application of shampoo into the hair and lather well.
- Wash all shampoo completely from the hair and scalp with warm tap water.
- Dry the hair thoroughly.

General advice
Avoid splashing shampoo into the eyes. If this occurs irrigate eyes immediately with normal saline or water.
Hair dryers should not be used when treating infected scalps; it is preferable to allow hair to dry naturally.
Towels, brushes and combs should not be shared.

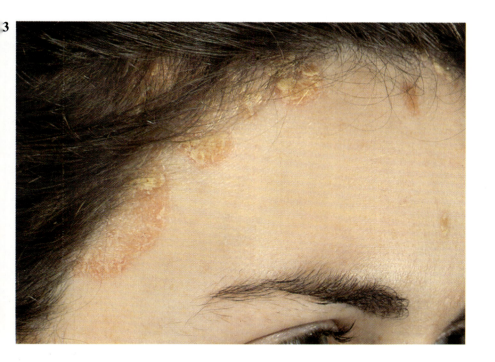

13

11 Tubular gauze—basic suit and adaptations

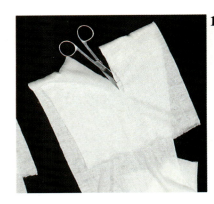

Uses

To reduce the spread and smearing of topical medication applied to skin lesions.
To keep the patient warm. Some inflammatory skin conditions can make the patient feel cold.
To cover unsightly lesions and make treatment more cosmetically acceptable.

Equipment

Tubular gauze (vest, arm and leg size).
Scissors.
Tray.

Procedure

A Vest
- Measure a length of large, vest-size, tubular gauze.
- Place flat on a clean surface.
- Overlap 20cm tubular gauze at the top. Cut a 20cm slit in the centre of the fold (Figure **14**).
- Fit the vest on to the patient (Figure **15**).

These measurements should be adapted to the patient's requirements.

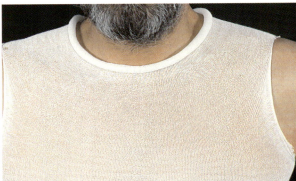

B Arms
- Measure a length of arm size tubular gauze.
- Feed the whole length on to your wrist.
- Hold the patient's hand with the nails protected by the palm of your hand.
- With your other hand (Figure **16**) feed the end of the dressing as far as the wrist. Withdraw your hand and take the gauze down to the top of the fingers. Double over the gauze and take remainder back to the wrist, feeding the total amount on to the patient's wrist. Cut holes in the end of the tubular gauze for the middle and little fingers (Figure **17**), and, slightly lower down, a hole for the thumb. Turn the hand over and cut a second hole for the middle finger, placing the latter through the hole to form a hand cover (Figure **18**). Take the gauze to the top of the arm and cut two slits in the top. Tie the slits to the vest by cutting two holes in the vest shoulders (Figure **19**).

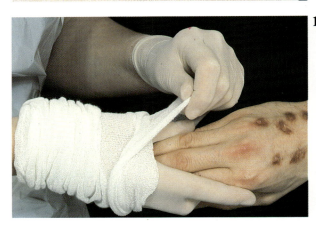

C Leg
- Measure a length of leg size tubular gauze.
- Feed the whole length on to your wrist.
- Holding the patient's toes in the palm of your hand to protect the nails (Figure **20**), feed the end of the dressing to the top of the ankle.

- Withdraw your hand slightly until the gauze is at the level of the toes.
- Twist the gauze once (Figure **21**) and take the gauze up the length of the leg.
- Cut two slits in the top of gauze and two complementary holes in the vest, and tie (Figure **22**).

Completed view (Figure **23**).

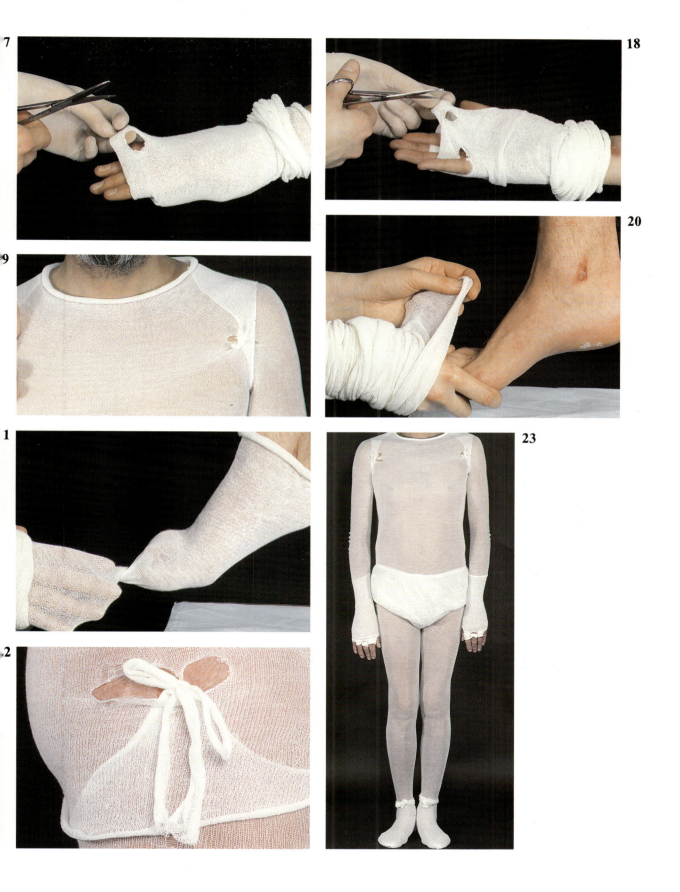

17

18

19

20

21

22

23

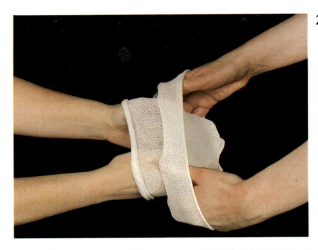

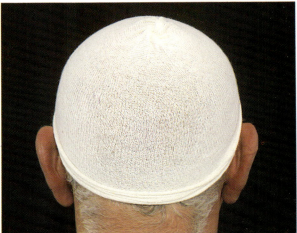

D Head Cover
- Cut a length of leg size tubular gauze approximately double the length of the head.
- One nurse holds the material over both splayed out hands.
- Another nurse twists the centre of the material and feeds the remainder back over the splayed out hands (Figure **24**).
- Remove the whole from the hands and place over the treated head (Figure **25**).

E Obesity vest
- Cut a double length of vest size tubular gauze to fit the patient.
- Cut down the whole length of one side of the gauze (Figure **26**).
- Flatten out the material.
- Fold the whole length in half and cut a 20cm slit across the material centre fold (Figure **27**).
- Place over the patient's head.
- Commencing at the axilla, sew the vest sides together (Figure **28**).

F Pants
- Cut a length of vest size tubular gauze, approximately double the lower abdominal length.
- One nurse holds half of the material over both splayed hands (Figure **29**).
- Another nurse twists the centre of the gauze and feeds the remainder over the gauze on the first nurse's hands.
- Cut two leg holes on either side (Figure **30**).
- Remove from the hands and fit on to the patient (Figure **31**).
- Tie at the waist by making a slit and tie the two halves together.
  Alternatively, thread a piece of stretched out tubular gauze through slits around the waist, draw together and tie.

G Powder Bag
- Cut 20cm of finger size tubular gauze.
- Knot one end of gauze to form a bag (Figure **32**).
- Fill a 20ml medicine pot with starch powder; empty powder into the gauze bag (Figure **33**).
- Twist the tubular gauze and fold it over the filled bag (Figure **34**).
- Knot this second layer on the top (Figure **35**).

General advice
Care should be taken not to smudge applied medication when fitting arm or leg tubular gauze, especially in the case of dithranol which may burn unaffected skin.

Tubular gauze stretches and may sag towards the end of the day.

Tubular gauze once applied, has come in contact with medications and numerous skin scales and, therefore, should not be used a second time, i.e. next day, as this can lead to cross infection. Fresh gauze should be used daily.

If hand and arm dressings are taken from the wrist to top of the arm before completing hand cover, there will be insufficient elasticity in the material to allow stretching over the fingers and this may catch the nails.

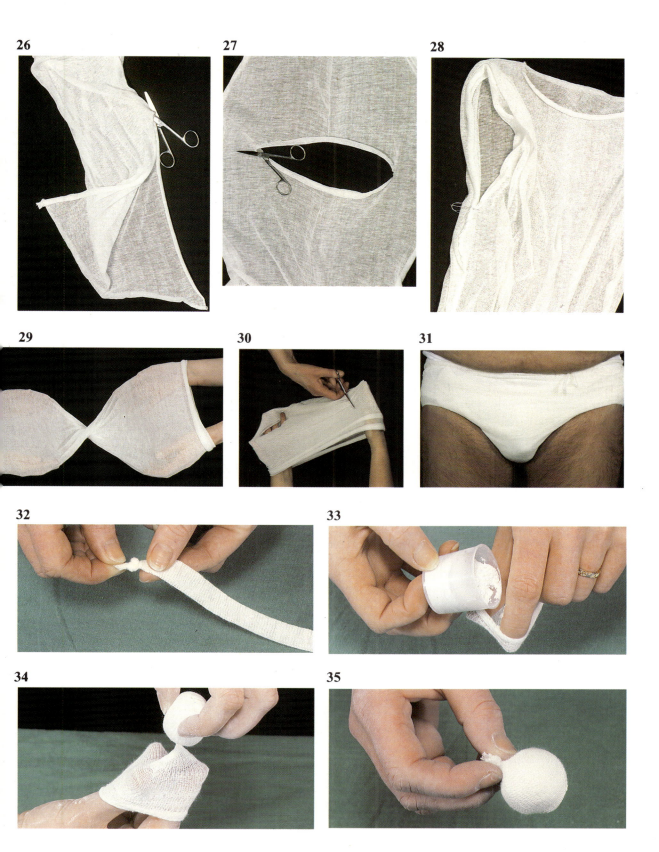

12   Dithranol (anthralin) application

Use
To treat psoriasis (Figure **36**). It is usually prescribed in three bases—
   paste: for large thick lesions.
   ointment/cream: for smaller lesions.

Equipment
Paper-lined tray containing:
   Prescribed medication.
   Prescription sheet with plastic cover.
   Wooden spatulae.
   Disposable gallipot.
   Disposable plastic apron.
   Disposable latex gloves.
   Disposable gallipot with starch powder bag.
   Disposable bag.
   Paper to cover seats and floor.
   Tubular gauze dressings.
   Scissors.

Procedure
N.B.   Patients often have tar baths and ultra-violet light (UVB) therapy prior to treatment with dithranol.

A In Lassar's paste

- Explain the procedure to patient.
- In a warm room, examine the total skin surface and record findings.
- Assess thickness of the lesion by feeling over the affected and surrounding unaffected skin with finger-tips.
- Position the patient comfortably.
- Don all protective clothing and cover seats and floor.
- Check medication against prescription.
- Decant a small quantity of paste into the gallipot, using a wooden spatula.
- Carefully apply dithranol to areas to be treated (Figure **37**), excluding any burnt areas from treatment.
- Using powder bag, dab starch powder on to treated areas to prevent spread of medication to normal skin (Figure **38**).
- Apply any prescribed ointment around treated lesions, to prevent burning.
- Apply tubular gauze covering to reduce smudging (Figure **39**).

B In Ointment/Cream Base

Follow same procedure as for dithranol in paste but rub medication into the skin lesions with a gloved hand (Figure **40**) and omit the use of starch powder.

Advice to nurse/patient
Treatment with dithranol may include a daily medicated bath and sometimes ultra-violet light exposure treatment.
Depending upon the skin response, daily treatment may take from 30 min.–4 hr., over 2–10 weeks.
Dithranol:
   can burn unaffected skin.
   stains skin and nails brown.
   stains clothing brown or purple.
   can stain light-coloured hair pink.

Short term contact treatment

Dithranol should be left on the skin for only 20 minutes of the prescribed time and then removed. Most patients find this both acceptable cosmetically and effective.
As dithranol treatment progresses, the initial low strength medication will be increased to a higher strength, usually every 2 days. To ensure that the skin will tolerate this on all lesions, the nurse will apply a small amount to a test area on a limb at 2-day intervals. Skin redness or soreness will indicate intolerance.
Dithranol should *never* be placed *near eyes*. If an accident occurs, wash eyes under running water for 20 minutes and seek medical aid.
If itching, redness, swelling, burning sensation or blistering of the skin occurs during treatment, remove medication with vegetable oil and bathe in plain water. Consult the doctor immediately.

Application of coal tar ointment

Psoriasis sometimes may be treated with coal tar ointment.
This may be applied over both affected and unaffected skin, remaining in place for 12-18 hours. It is usually given in conjunction with ultra-violet light therapy.

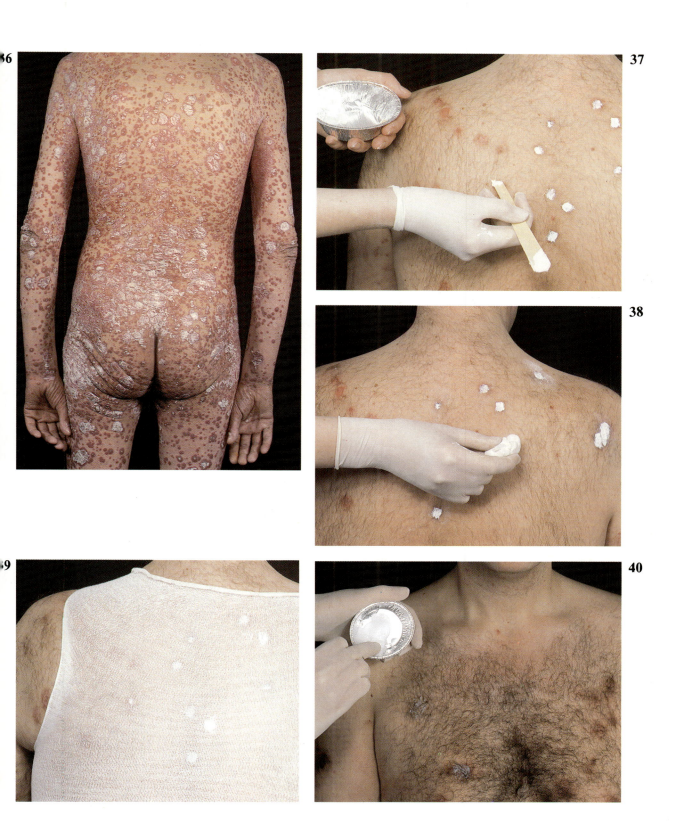

13 Polythene occlusion

Use
To clear thick skin lesions or lesions not responding to other treatment.

Equipment
Paper-lined tray containing:
    Prescribed medication.
    Polythene square or self-adherent polythene film.
    Foil tray containing:
        Gallipot
        Wooden spatula
        Tubular gauze as required.
    Plastic apron.
    Latex gloves.
    Paper cover.
    Paper adhesive tape.
    Sterile non-adherent gauze, if required.

Procedure
- Apply prescribed medication with a gloved hand to the affected area (Figure **41**).
- Place polythene around the limb (Figure **42**).
- Two pieces of sterile non-adherent gauze may be placed under the polythene at each end to absorb excess moisture (Figure **43**). If the foot is occluded, four pieces of gauze placed between the toes will absorb excess moisture.
- Tape the ends of the occlusion leaving a 1–2.5cm margin at each end to accomodate any accumulating oedema (Figure **44**).
- Apply tubular gauze over the polythene and tie with a loose knot (Figure **45**). If the foot is being treated cover with a double gauze sock.

Advice to nurse/patient
Polythene occlusion encourages increased medication absorption through soggy keratin and should be used only on prescription.
Polythene occlusion should be changed daily.
Treatment usually lasts for 3–4 days.
If any skin discomfort occurs, contact the doctor immediately.

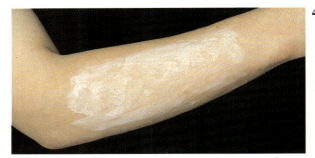

4

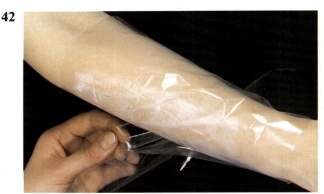

42

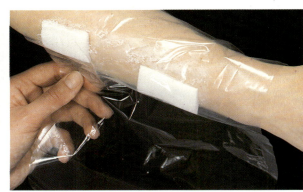

4

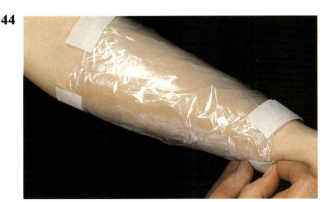

44

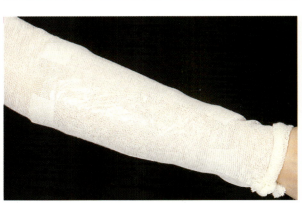

4

14   Care of the erythrodermic patient

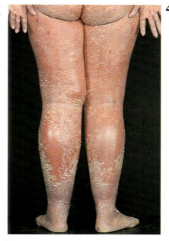

46

**Procedure should be used only in hospital, under
medical supervision.**

Erythroderma is a state of generalised redness of
the skin, usually due to a flare-up of a pre-existing
skin condition, e.g. erythrodermic psoriasis
(Figure **46**).
The aim of nursing care is to reduce heat, fluid
and protein loss from the skin surface.

Advice to nurse
Place the patient in a separate cubicle to rest
and to avoid infection.
Check that room temperature is a constant 80^0F
(26^0C), with more heating available, if possible.
Record temperature, pulse, respiration and
general condition 4-hourly.
Fluid balance should be maintained and an
accurate fluid intake and output chart kept and
monitored regularly, to avoid dehydration.
Passive physiotherapy and deep breathing
exercises are given three times a day.
Twice-weekly bacteriological swabs may be
taken from various areas of the skin—the nose,
throat, axillae, umbilicus and any moist areas
are the most useful.
The skin may be red, swollen and tender. It
may be broken and wet in many parts.
Give regular analgesia as prescribed, if
necessary.
Food should be served attractively in small
amounts maintaining a balanced diet.
A bed bath or normal bath may be given as
prescribed, taking care to prevent chilling.
An optimistic approach is essential in order to
encourage the patient.

Equipment
Paper-lined tray containing:
Prescription sheet, covered with polythene.
Prescribed medication.
Non-adherent dressings.
Bandages or tubular gauze.
Disposable latex gloves.
Disposable plastic apron.
Disposable gallipot.
Disposable bag.
Wooden spatula.
Non-adherent sheet.

Procedure
- Explain procedure to the patient.
- Ensure adequate analgesia.
- Take tray to patient.

- Don plastic apron and latex gloves.
- Check medication against prescription.
- Decant medication into gallipot.
- Spread medication on to non-adherent
  dressing surface with wooden spatula.
- Apply non-adherent dressings to the skin. This
  reduces the pain sometimes experienced when
  raw skin surface is touched.
- Hold dressings in place with bandages or
  tubular gauze.
- Position patient on a non-adherent sheet,
  sitting up to maintain respiratory function.
- Dispose of all materials and cleanse tray.

Special advice to nurse
Turn patient regularly to prevent the occurrence
of pressure sores. The patient may benefit from
the use of a special bed such as a temperature-
controlled microsphere flotation bed, where the
patient floats on a bed of fluidised beads.
The advantages include:
– high prevention of pressure sores
– greater maintenance of body heat
– easing of discomfort, which may help to reduce
  the need for, or quantity of medication for pain
  relief
– absorbtion of any excessive exudate
– may help to increase the rate of healing of the
  skin.

Advice to patient
Always mention any concerns about your
condition or treatment to the nurse or doctor.
Do not be afraid to ask for anything you require.
Treatment lasts for about 2–10 weeks depending
upon the response of the skin.

15   Wet wraps

Procedure should be used only in hospital, under medical supervision.

Use
To re-hydrate skin affected with some types of eczema e.g. generalised dry, flaking eczema (Figure **47**).

Equipment
Lint square 25cm × 25cm.
Freshly laundered bath towels.
Bowl of warm water.
Polythene pillow case *or* polythene sheet.
Cotton pillow case *or* cotton sheet.

Procedure
A Face wraps

- Explain procedure to the patient.
- Check that room temperature is at least 80^{0}F (26^{0}C).
- Check patient's temperature and examine the total skin surface to be treated.
- Cut a lint mask to size.
- Draw a paper stencil of mask and place in treatment notes for use next day.
- Cover pillow with polythene pillow case and a towel.
- Position patient comfortably with head on towel.
- Apply cream to face as prescribed.
- Cover face with lint mask wrung out in warm water (Figure **48**).
- Leave for prescribed length of time, re-soaking mask in warm water if lint is drying out.
- Remove mask and *immediately* apply prescribed ointment.

B Limb wraps and total body wraps
- Explain procedure to the patient.
- Check that room temperature is at least 80^{0}F (26^{0}C).
- Check patient's temperature and examine the total area of skin to be treated.
- Prepare bed with polythene sheet and lay undressed patient on bed.
- Apply prescribed cream to the affected areas (Figure **49**).
- Cover limbs/body with towels wrung out in warm water (Figures **50, 51**).
- Place two blankets over areas being treated, to reduce chilling.
- Check frequently, re-soaking wraps in warm water, if they are drying out.
- Leave for prescribed length of time.
- Remove wraps and *immediately* apply prescribed ointment.
- Check patient's temperature and allow him to rest comfortably, fully dressed.

General advice
Wet wraps treatment is suitable for only a few eczema patients. Wet cloth around the skin can reduce body temperature rapidly and may induce hypothermia, therefore it should be used only as a hospital treatment.
If any discomfort occurs, contact the doctor immediately.

N.B.   No loose polythene should be used when a child is being treated; suffocation can result if a child is restless or sedated.

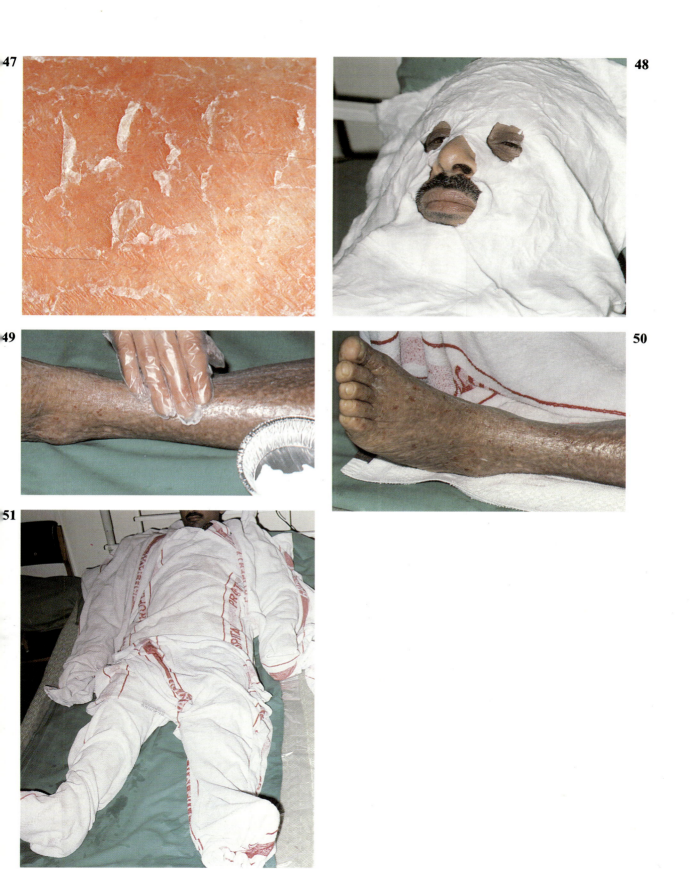

16   Dressing technique in generalised body ulceration

Procedure should be used only in hospital, under medical supervision.

Equipment
Paper-lined tray containing:
Prescription sheet covered with polythene.
Prescribed medication.
Bacteriological swab, if required.
Tubular gauze dressings.
Cotton bandages.
Paper adhesive tape.
Non-adherent dressings.
Wooden spatulae.
Disposable plastic apron.
Disposable latex gloves.
Disposal bag.

Procedure
- Don the plastic apron and latex gloves.
- Prepare tray dressings.
- Apply prescribed medication to the dressing surface, using spatula to spread evenly (Figure 52).
- Form a stack of prepared dressings in the tray, placing prepared surface (Figure 53).
- To prepare the vest, cut a 20cm length in the middle of a double (vest-size) large tubular gauze measured to fit the patient (Figure 54).
- To prepare each sleeve, cut a 20cm slit through one layer of the tubular gauze at the top of the width (Figure 55) and a 40cm slit through one layer of tubular gauze at the bottom of the width. The centre of this cut is half the length of the material.
- Explain the procedure to the patient.
- Before commencing treatment, take any swabs required for pathological investigations.
- Ease the large gauze vest to the waist; avoid touching the skin, thus preventing pain and cross infection.
  If arms are ulcerated it may be necessary to take the gauze over the lower limbs; avoid touching the skin (Figure 56).
- Position the non-adherent dressing in place with the edges close together. Avoid moving dressings once in place as this can cause pain (Figures 57, 58).
- When the whole trunk is covered (Figure 59), tie the corners of the vest. Knots can cause pressure and pain. In severe conditions an extra shoulder dressing may be required to cushion the knots against the skin. Axillae dressings are secured in the vest top.

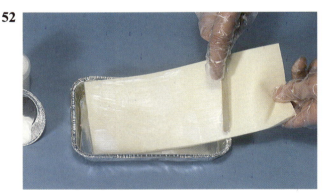

52

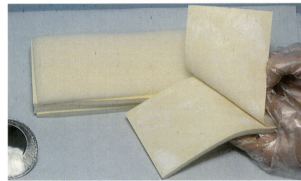

53

54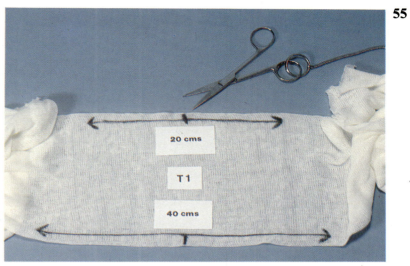

T2   20 cms

55

20 cms

T1

40 cms

56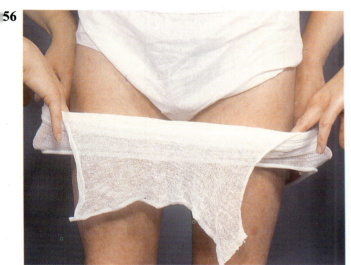

57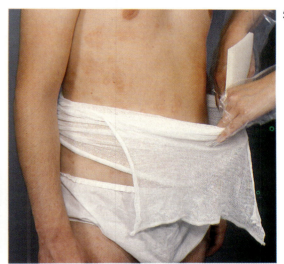

58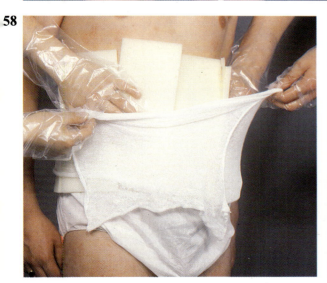

59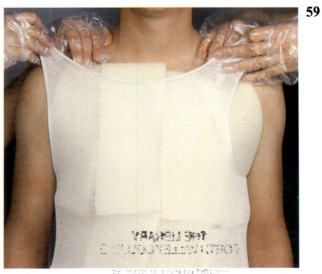

29

- Dress the arms avoiding the use of tape (Figure **60**), as this tends to cause epidermal stripping as it is removed.
- Tuck end of axillae dressings into the gauze with 1cm sleeve end and 1cm vest end (Figure **61**).
- Place arm dressing over the head (Figures **62, 63**) with the 20cm cut at the top and the 40cm cut at the bottom and put patient's arms through the sleeves.
- Cut wrist end of the dressing and tie around wrist (Figures **64, 65**).
- Dress leg lesions (Figure **66**).

- Feed dressing on to your own wrist and hold patient's toes (Figure **67**). Covering the nails with the palm of your hand to protect them against snagging, as jagged nails may catch on the gauze side. (The use of metal frames for gauze application may cause pain.)
- Feed dressing end up to the ankle and twist remainder once around the great toe (Figure **68**), feeding the dressing back over the foot up to the top of the leg.
- Tie by making complementary cuts and slits in the gauze of the vest bottom and leg tops (Figure **69**).

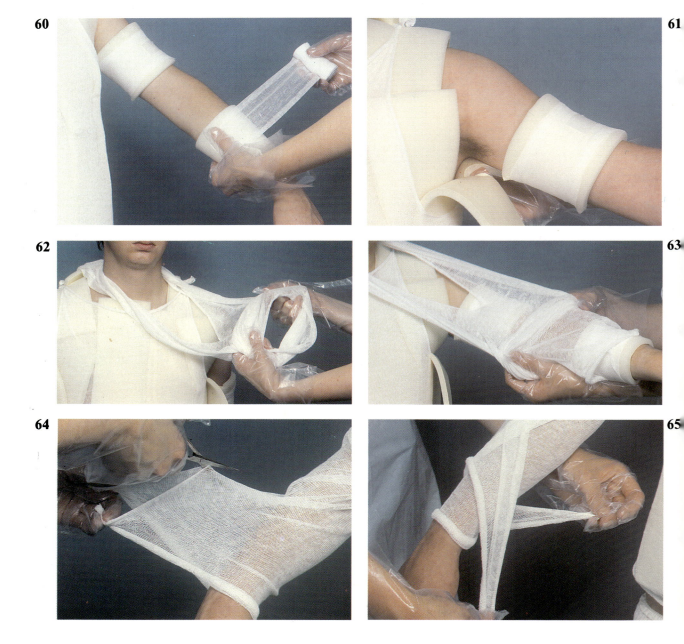

60

61

62

63

64

65

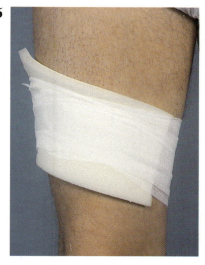

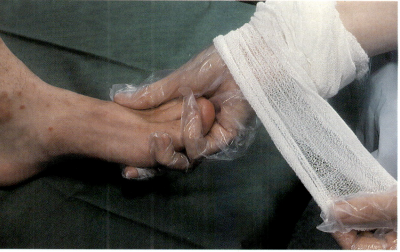

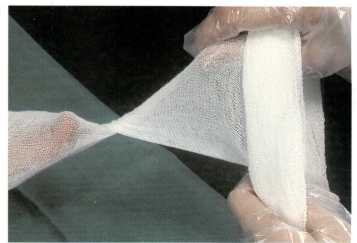

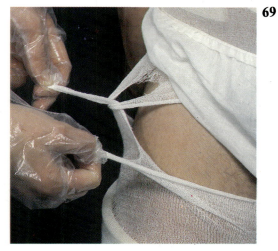

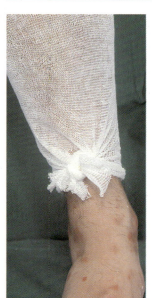

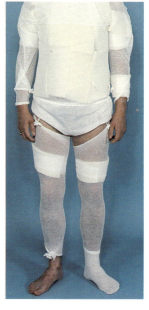

- Dressings can be tied at the ankle, leaving two finger-widths of space between the leg and material to prevent oedema (Figures **70**, **71**).

N.B. Patients with generalised body ulceration or generalised pustular psoriasis usually benefit from the use of a special bed such as a temperature-controlled microsphere flotation bed (see page 38).

Advice to patient
Advantages of this dressing technique:
reduces heat, fluid and protein loss from the body;
increases mobility and ability to exercise as the dressings are well secured;
pain is often relieved when ulcers are occluded.

17 Aspiration of blisters in generalised bullous eruption

Procedure should be used only in hospital, under medical supervision.

Uses

To reduce discomfort in generalised blistering skin conditions, e.g. pemphigus, pemphigoid.
To allow accurate recording of fluid loss from blisters.
To prevent cross infection between blisters.

Equipment

Paper-lined tray containing:
Prescription chart covered in polythene.
Prescribed medication.
Medicine pot (60ml).
Universal containers 2–4.
Sterile scissors (e.g. Iris scissors).
10ml syringe × 4 as required.
23 gauge sterile needle × 10.
Sterile gauze (2 packs).
Sterile latex gloves.
Non-adherent dressings.
Cotton bandages and tape.
Tubular gauze cut to size.
Disposable plastic apron.
Disposable latex gloves.
Disposable gallipot.
Disposal bag.
Wooden spatula.
Socially clean cotton gown.
Fresh clothing for patient.
Paper square.

Procedure

- Ensure adequate analgesia.
- Check that room temperature is approx. 75⁰–80⁰F (24⁰–26⁰C).
- Explain procedure to patient.
- Don plastic apron and cover with socially clean gown.
- Stand undressed patient on paper square.
- Count number of unbroken blisters on skin surface and record result. It is useful to divide limbs and body into sections visually to avoid miscounting.
- Note any apparently infected blisters and treat these last.
- Don sterile gloves.
- Starting with the trunk, aspirate fluid from the blister into a 10ml syringe. Insert the needle into the top edge of the blister to prevent fluid dripping down the syringe (Figure **72**). Point the needle, bevel uppermost, towards the painless roof of the blister (Figure **73**).

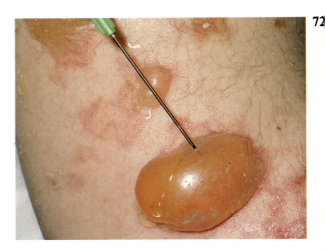

72

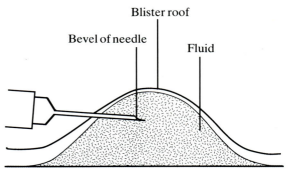

7.

Bevel of needle — Blister roof — Fluid

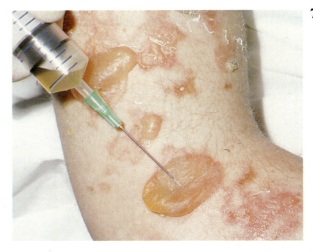

7

- Aspirate until blister collapses, leaving a small amount of fluid *in situ* to prevent pulling of the two skin surfaces, as this would cause pain (Figure **74**).
- Gently lift the roof of the collapsed blister; with sterile scissors, cut out a section and soak up remaining fluid with sterile gauze.
- Continue until all the apparently non-infected blisters have been treated.
- Proceed with the apparently infected blisters. A change of needle will be required for various areas of the body, i.e. one for the upper arm and one for the lower arm.
- Blister fluid should be measured into a medicine pot.
- Two or three measured quantities in sterile containers are sent for bacterial culture and sensitivity screening.
- Change sterile latex gloves for disposable latex gloves.
- (a) A bath may have been prescribed to dry the skin lesions when procedure is completed.
- (b) If not, decant a small quantity of medication into a gallipot and check it against the prescription. Spread medication, with a spatula on to the non-adherent dressing surface.
- Apply dressing to lesions to be treated and bandage in place. Cover with tubular gauze for extra support.
- Position patient comfortably.
- Measure fluid loss and record on fluid intake/output chart.
- Dispose of materials, checking that all syringes and needles are accounted for.
- Record all findings in patient's notes.

Advice to nurse/patient
It is important that the patient should rest after procedure.
Regular intake and output of fluids will be recorded on a chart.
New blisters will be counted daily.

N.B. Plastic aprons are covered with a gown to prevent adherence of plastic to the wet skin surface if the two are inadvertently statically adhered.
Latex gloves, unlike plastic, do not adhere to fragile blistered skin.

18 Application of impregnated adhesive tapes

Use
To apply medication under occlusion over a period of time to, e.g. lichen planus and keloids.

Equipment
Prescribed impregnated (usually with a corticosteroid) tape.
Adhesive tape.
Scissors.

Procedure
- Explain procedure to the patient.
- Position patient comfortably and expose area to be treated (Figure **75**).
- Cut impregnated tape to the size of the lesion to be covered.
- Apply impregnated tape directly on to the lesion (Figure **76**).
- Cover tape with a strip of adhesive tape.

Advice to patient
Use the tape only as prescribed.
Apply impregnated tape exactly to the lesion.
Change impregnated tape once every 24 hours or according to instructions. The lesion should be left exposed to rest the skin for a few hours between applications of the impregnated adhesive tape.

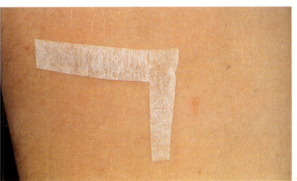

75

76

19   Application of medicated paste bandages

Use
To help to control irritation, inflammation or lichenification, particularly in eczema (Figures **77, 78**).

Equipment
Prescribed cotton gauze medicated paste bandage (impregnated with, e.g. zinc, calamine, tar).
Tubular cotton gauze bandage.
Tubular elasticated bandage.
Adhesive tape.

Procedure
- Explain procedure to the patient.
- Position the patient comfortably.
- Check that the patient is not allergic to the dressing to be used.
- Begin bandaging at the wrist (Figure **79**) or the foot (Figure **80**).
- After each turn around the limb, cut or fold the bandage and apply in the opposite direction. This aids removal and also avoids circulation problems if the limb becomes oedematous.
- Fold and reverse the bandage (Figures **81, 82**), or cut on each turn until the area to be treated has been covered (Figure **83**).
- Use tubular gauze to fix bandages in place, thus reducing the risk of damage to fragile skin. It is difficult to apply conventional bandages with an even pressure and any ridges can cause further damage to the affected skin area (Figures **84, 85**).

77
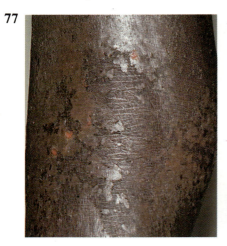

78
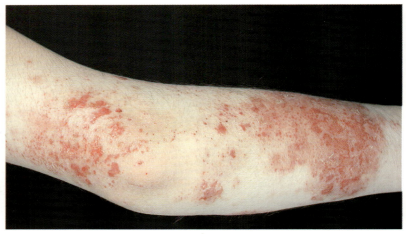

79
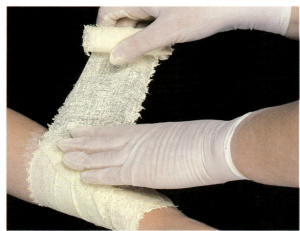

80
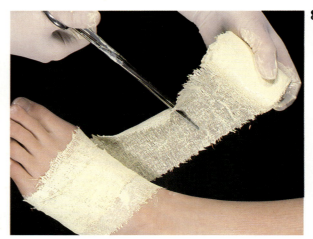

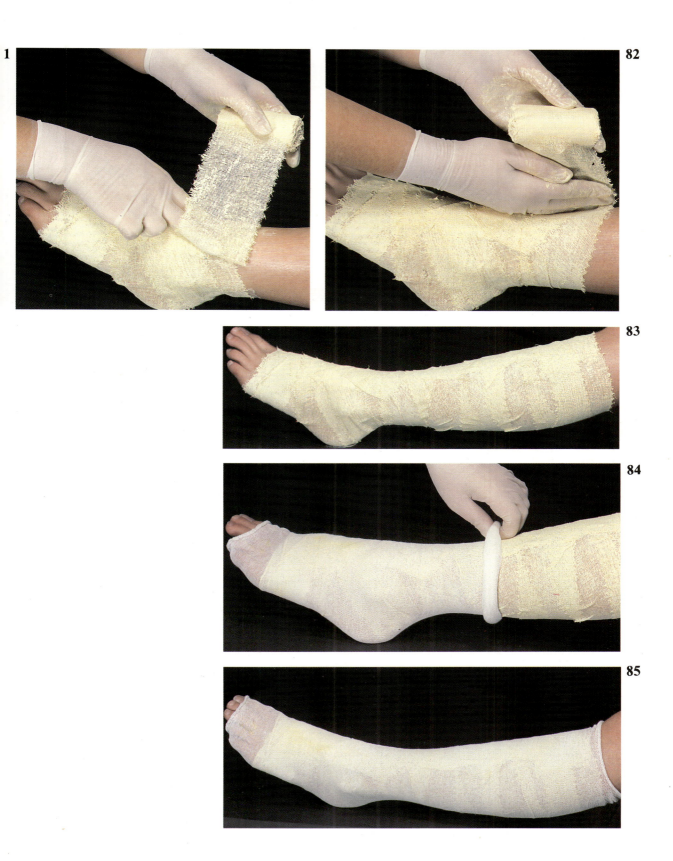

- Apply elasticated tubular bandage over the top of the dressing (Figure **86**). Fix adhesive elastic tape at each end to prevent the edges from rolling (Figure **87**). This protects the medicated bandage, keeps it in place and discourages the patient from scratching.

General advice
Keep the dressing dry.
The bandage should be kept in place for the length of time prescribed by the doctor; this may be up to a week.

If the limb becomes grossly oedematous/swollen, the bandages should be removed and the doctor informed.

Advice to patient
In cases where the medicated paste bandage is only left on overnight, it may be advisable to apply a self-adherent wrap bandage directly over the medicated paste bandage, instead of using tubular bandages (Figures **88, 89**). This alternative method may be preferable, particularly with children.

86

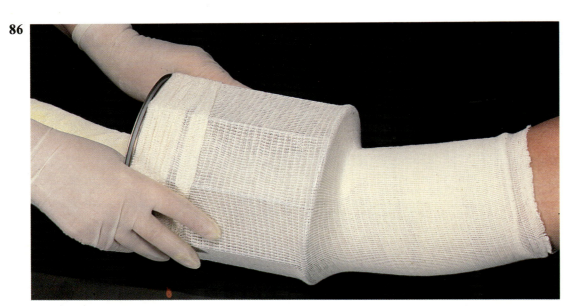

87

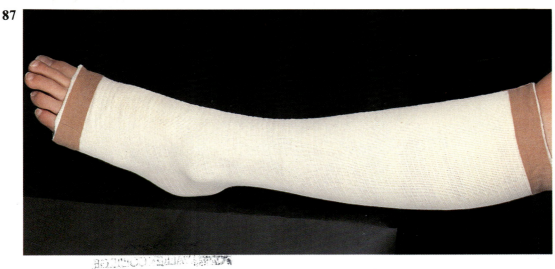

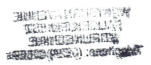

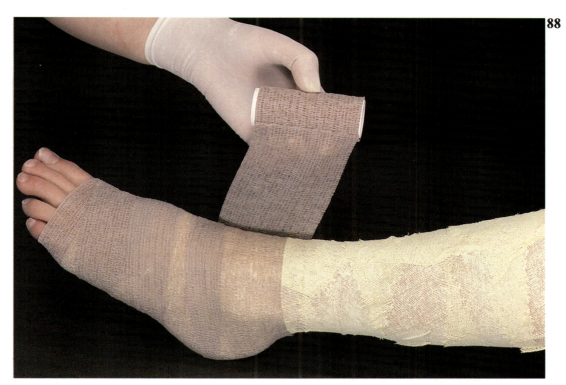

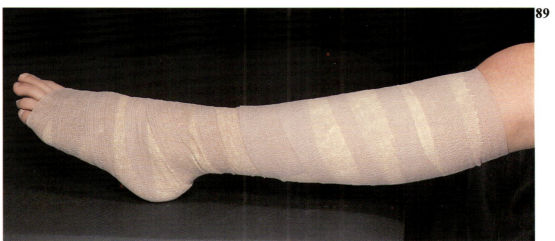

20 Emollients and moisturisers

Uses
- To re-hydrate the skin.
- soften dry, cracked skin.
- To help to keep the skin supple and retain its moisture.

Equipment
Pot of emulsifying ointment.
Wooden spatula.
Gallipot.
Hot tap water.

Procedure
- Using the wooden spatula, decant a small quantity of emulsifying ointment into the gallipot.
- Add 2–3ml hot tap water.
- With the wooden spatula, stir until well mixed and creamy, adding a little more water if required.
- Using small quantities on each area, apply the ointment to the dry surface of the skin in the direction of the hair fall. This avoids the ointment becoming trapped in the hair base and the possible growth of bacteria.

General advice
Emollients can be applied as many times as required but avoid clogging the skin pores by thick applications.

Use an emollient when the skin is dry and no longer inflamed.

Avoid the unnecessary use of prescribed medication on non-inflamed but dry skin, in order to prevent another outbreak of inflammation; use an emollient instead.

All medications applied to the skin are absorbed into the body. If medication is applied to a non-inflamed area, the body is exposed to more medication than required, thus lessening its effectiveness if it is prescribed again.

dispose of any unused emollient that has been made into a cream; it will grow bacteria if exposed to air.

A supple skin will discourage the formation of painful, dry cracks. Experience will show the quantity of moisturiser to apply to the skin.

It is preferable to avoid perfumed moisturisers as they can cause an adverse reaction in some individuals.

Use of emollients
Common emollients or moisturisers (e.g. emulsifying ointment BP, aqueous cream BP, '50:50' equal parts of liquid paraffin and white soft paraffin) may be used in various ways.

Prior to bathing or showering, dab on to the skin in dots (Figure **90**), then spread the emollient over the body, stroking gently in the direction of the hair fall (Figure **91**).

As moisturiser
Smooth on to the skin immediately after bathing. Apply as often as needed to prevent skin becoming dry.

As cleanser
Apply liberally to the skin and wipe off gently with a single layer of paper tissue, taking care not to damage fragile skin (Figure **92**).

As a soap substitute
Mix emollient with water in the palm to form a lather (Figure **93**).
Smooth on to skin in the same way as soap.
Gently rinse lather off skin.
Pat dry.

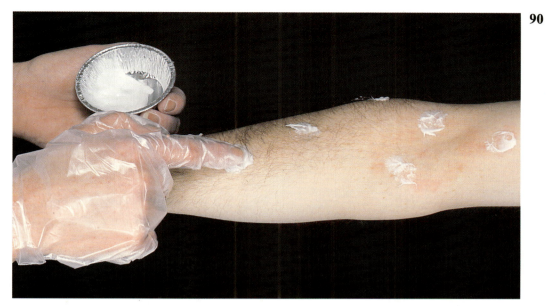

90

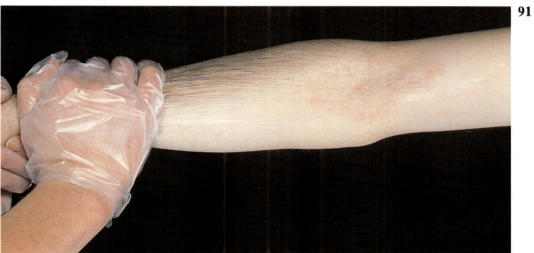

91

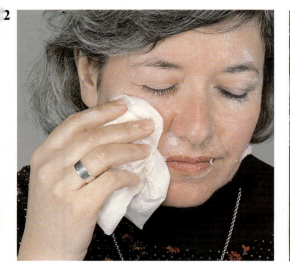

2

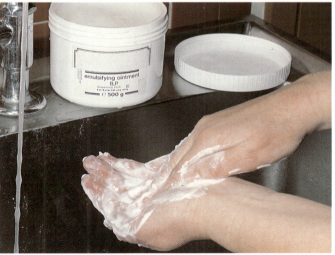

93

21 Removal of nails with urea

Urea ointment is applied to the nails which are infected with *Trichophyton rubrum* or *Candida albicans*.

Use
To soften the nails in preparation for removal.

Equipment
Tray containing:
 Tincture of benzoin compound.
 Elastic adhesive tape, 2.5cm width.
 Cotton wool swab stick.
 Cotton tubular bandage, 1.5cm width.
 Self-adherent polythene film.
 Urea ointment as prescribed.
 Scissors.
 Tubular bandage applicator.
 Wooden spatula.

Procedure
- Explain procedure to the patient.
- Position patient comfortably.
- Check that the patient is not allergic to elastic adhesive tape; if so, substitute a non-allergenic tape.
- Paint the skin around the nail with tincture of benzoin compound (Figure **94**).
- Cut two lengths of elastic adhesive tape and apply over the tincture around the nail to protect surrounding skin (Figure **95**).
- Apply the urea ointment generously to the nail *only* (Figure **96**).
- Occlude the nail with polythene film (Figures **97**, **98**) and secure the whole of the occlusion with the elastic adhesive tape (Figure **99**).
- Cover this dressing with another layer of polythene film and secure (Figure **100**).
- Apply cotton tubular bandage over finger or toe and fix in place with elastic adhesive bandage (Figure **101**).
- Keep dressing *in situ* for 1–2 weeks; the nail should then be soft enough for removal by the doctor.

Advice to patient
Keep dressing dry.
If any severe discomfort occurs, contact the doctor.

94

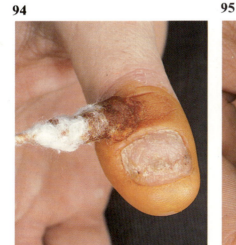

95

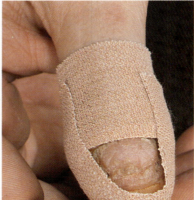

96

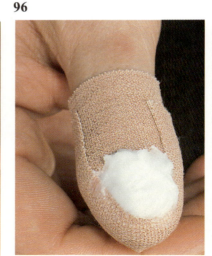

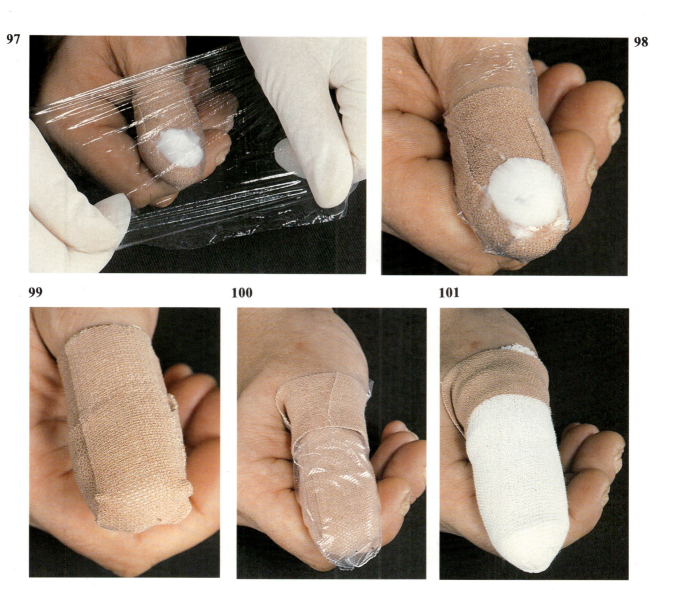

22 Nail care in psoriasis

Use
To avoid damage of affected nails and to maintain cosmetically acceptable nails.

Equipment
Emery board and nail file.
Nail clippers.

Advice to patient
Keep nails short and well-manicured to prevent them from catching and separating from the nail bed.

Wherever possible, it is preferable to file nails rather than cut them, as this avoids excessive trauma to the nail.

Always file nails from above (Figure **102**). This avoids pressure under the nail (Figure **103**) which could cause it to separate from the nail bed.

Care should be taken to avoid damage to the cuticle; this may provide an entry site for infection.

Correct

102

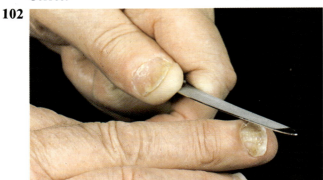

Incorrect

10

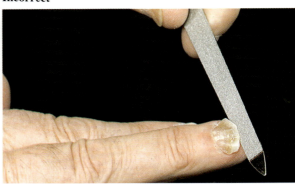

23 Comedone (blackhead) extraction

Uses
May be necessary in some patients with cystic acne.
Cosmetic, although of temporary benefit (Figure **104**).

Equipment
Light.
Magnifying lens.
Alcohol-impregnated swabs.
Comedone extractor.
Latex gloves.

Procedure
- Explain procedure to the patient and reassure throughout.
- Position the patient comfortably.
- Apply warm compress to face for a few minutes.
- Clean the site with an alcohol swab.
- Gently express the comedone through the hole of the extractor (Figure **105**) and remove (Figure **106**).
- Wipe the site with a fresh alcohol swab.

Advice to patient
Keep hands away from face.
Keep hair off face—wash hair daily if necessary.
Continue treatment prescribed by the doctor.

104

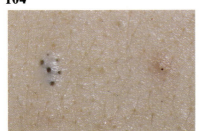

105

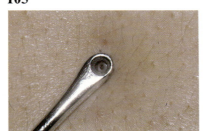

106

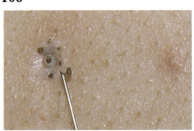

24   Milia (keratin cyst) extraction

Use
Cosmetic (Figure **107**).

Equipment
Alcohol-impregnated swabs.
Sterile needle, large gauge.
Latex gloves.

Procedure
- Explain procedure to the patient and reassure throughout.
- Position the patient lying down comfortably.
- Clean the skin with an alcohol swab, taking care near the eyes.
- Break the epidermis over the cyst using a sterile needle (Figure **108**); lift out the cyst on the end of the needle (Figure **109**).
- Wipe the site with a fresh alcohol swab.

Advice to patient
Keep hands away from face.
Gently pat area dry after washing.

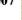
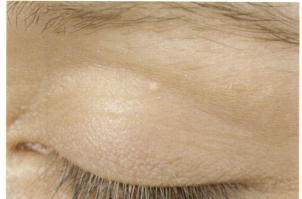
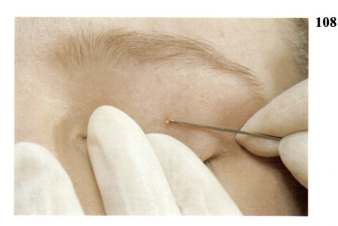

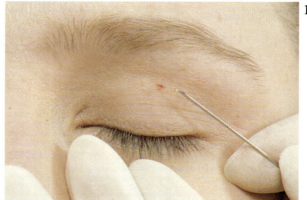

25 Paring viral warts

Use
To improve the effectiveness of warts treatment applications.

Equipment
'Corn and callus' remover.
Scalpel—if paring plantar warts.
Paper tissue.
Pumice stone.

Procedure
- Explain procedure to the patient.
- Position patient comfortably sitting or lying down.
- Rub away surface of wart with pumice stone or corn remover.

- If skin over wart becomes thick and hard (Figure **110**), (as frequently occurs during the course of treatment), pare the wart carefully with a scalpel (Figure **111**), until the thrombosed vessel ends are visible as 'black dots' in the wart (Figure **112**).
- Dispose of paper tissue containing pared skin.

Advice to patient
Always pare the wart surface before treatment application. If this is done before every treatment, a 'corn remover' is usually adequate to remove the wart surface. Avoid cutting into the wart as this can cause pain and bleeding.

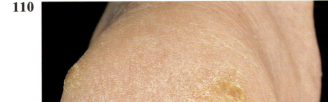

110

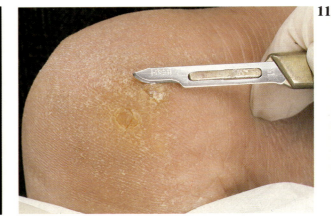

11

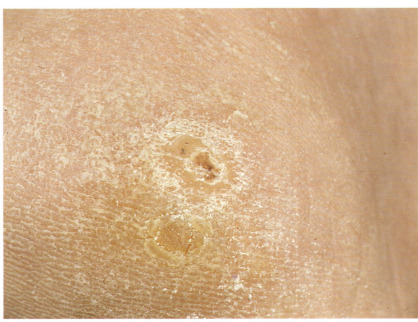

112

26 Treatment of warts with salicylic acid plaster

Use
To treat plantar viral warts, corns.

Equipment
Salicylic acid plaster.
Adhesive plaster.
Corn remover.
Hot water.

Procedure
- Soak foot in hot water for at least 5 minutes, (e.g. during a bath) and then dry.
- Pare surface of the wart.

- Cut salicylic acid plaster to size of the wart and apply exactly to cover the lesion (Figure **113**).
- Fix in place with adhesive plaster (Figure **114**).
- Repeat procedure every 1–3 days; macerated keratin will separate.

Advice to patient
If the foot becomes painful, stop treatment and consult the doctor.
If treatment is carried out correctly and regularly, most warts should be cured in about 12 weeks.

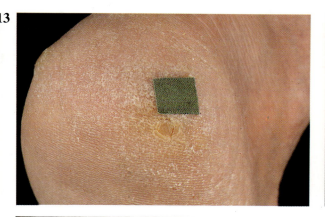

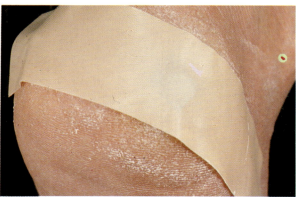

27 Treatment of warts with podophyllum resin

Use
To treat mainly anogenital warts (Figure **115**).

Equipment
Tray containing:
Podophyllum resin preparation as prescribed.
Starch powder.
Cotton wool swab sticks.
Petroleum jelly.
Disposable latex glove.

Procedure
- Explain procedure to the patient.
- Position the patient comfortably and expose the area to be treated.
- Protect skin surrounding wart with petroleum jelly.
- Dip cotton wool swab stick in podophyllum preparation.
- Apply preparation precisely on to wart.
- Shake starch powder on to treated wart.
- Wash the preparation off after 6–8 hours.

N.B. Podophyllum treatment must not be used on facial warts or during pregnancy. Warts often extend into the anus or vagina, if this occurs, consult the doctor.

Advice to patient
Treatment should be carried out weekly.
If severe burning occurs after treatment, the podophyllum preparation should be washed off immediately.
If severe adverse reaction develops, stop treatment and consult the doctor.

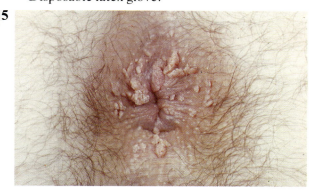

28   Treatment of warts with formaldehyde soaks

Use
To treat plantar viral warts.

Equipment
Tray containing:
  Formaldehyde solution as prescribed.
  Shallow container (e.g. small saucer).
  Petroleum jelly.
  Paper towel.
  Warm water.

Procedure
- Explain procedure to the patient.
- Position patient comfortably with the foot well supported.
- Pour a small amount of formaldehyde solution into the container.
- Protect the unaffected skin around the wart with petroleum jelly (Figure **116**).

- Place only the affected part of the foot in the formaldehyde solution (Figure **117**), supporting the rest of the foot in a comfortable position.
- Soak wart for 10 minutes.
- Dry skin with the paper towel to remove any residual formaldehyde solution.
- Bathe foot in warm water.

Advice to patient
Pare off any dry skin before treatment; if this is done immediately after treatment, it may cause stinging and discomfort.
Treatment should be carried out twice daily.
If the foot becomes very sore, leave for 2–3 days before paring.
If treatment is carried out correctly, most warts should be cured within 12 weeks.

116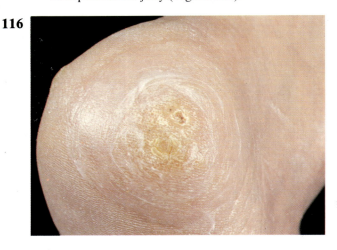

11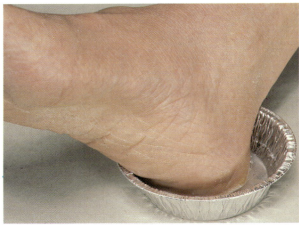

---

29   Treatment of warts with liquid nitrogen

Use
To treat viral warts (verrucas) (Figure **118**).

Equipment
  Flask of liquid nitrogen *or* liquid nitrogen spray.
  Cotton wool swab stick.
  Adhesive plaster.

Procedure
- Explain procedure to the patient.
- Position patient comfortably.
- Dip swab stick into liquid nitrogen until cotton wool is frozen.
  or Spray liquid nitrogen directly on to wart.

- Apply frozen cotton wool tip to wart (Figure **119**).
— for small warts on thin skin, treat for 5–10 seconds.
— for large warts on thick skin, (e.g. soles, palms), treat for 15–30 seconds.
- Cover treated lesions with adhesive plaster.

N.B. Take care not to burn normal skin when applying liquid nitrogen which is -190^{0}C.

Advice to patient
A blister with the wart in the roof usually forms

within 2 days. If this remains intact, the area need not be covered.
If the blister becomes large, tense and painful, it may be pricked with a needle which has been sterilised in a flame and a simple dry dressing applied.

Pain can be controlled easily with a simple analgesic.
At least one week must elapse between treatments, even if a blister does not form.
If a treated area becomes infected or extremely painful consult the doctor.

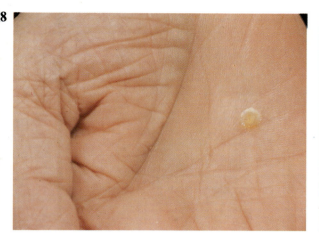
8

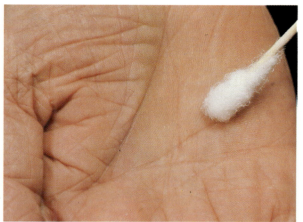
119

30   Treatment of warts with salicylic acid collodion

Use
To treat viral warts on hands.

Equipment
  Salicylic acid collodion.
  Sharpened orange stick.

Procedure
- Explain procedure to the patient.
- Ensure patient washes hands thoroughly with soap and water.
- Apply salicylic acid preparation carefully to wart with orange stick (Figure **120**). Avoid painting normal skin.
- Allow to dry.

Advice to patient
Repeat treatment each night. If it is carried out correctly and regularly, most warts should be cured within 12 weeks.
Check with the doctor at intervals.
Keep bottle of preparation tightly closed.

N.B. Do not apply treatment to any warts that have been frozen with liquid nitrogen until the inflammation has subsided.

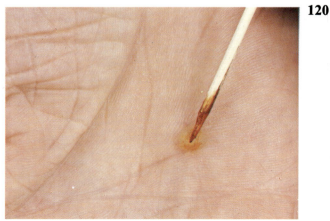
120

31 Removal of crusts

Use
To remove crusts on lesions, e.g. impetigo (Figure **121**), prior to treatment.

Equipment
Tray containing:
  Gauze swab.
  Antiseptic solution in gallipot.
  Disposable paper towel.
  Disposable plastic sheet.
  Latex gloves.
  Starch poultice.
  Sterile forceps.

Procedure
- Explain procedure to the patient and reassure throughout.
- Position patient comfortably and expose the area to be treated.
- Protect patient's clothing with a plastic sheet and paper towel. Put on gloves.
- With swabs soaked in antiseptic solution, moisten the crust until it is soft.
- Gently remove the softened crust, taking care not to damage any surrounding skin or hair follicles. Use sterile forceps to lift the crust if necessary.
- When the crust has been removed, gently dry the area.
- If starch poultice is used, apply to the lesion until the crust is soft enough for gentle removal.

Advice to patient
Keep the lesion areas crust-free.
Apply a covering dressing if necessary.

121

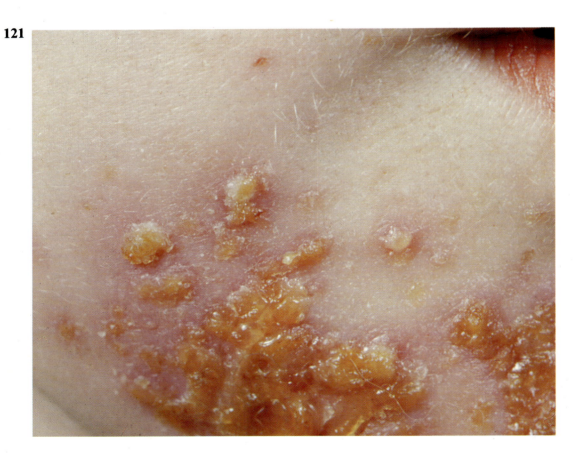

32 Topical skin care in acne

A Abrasives and keratolytics

Use
To peel off the superficial layers of the skin and unblock the openings of the pilosabaceous follicles in mild and moderate acne (Figure **122**).

Equipment
Soap.
Water.
Prescribed medication.

Procedure

Abrasives
- Wash face gently, rinse well to remove soap.
- Apply prescribed medication to wet skin as instructed. Take care to avoid the eyes.
- Rinse well and pat dry.

Keratolytics
- Wash face gently, pat dry.
- Apply prescribed medication as instructed (usually once or twice daily). Take care to avoid the eyes.

Advice to patient
Excessive irritation and dryness may occur, especially during the first few weeks of treatment. This may be relieved by reducing the frequency of application and using a moisturiser.

B Topical vitamin A acid

Use
To clear keratin plugs from follicular ducts in more severe acne.

Equipment
Prescribed medication.

Procedure
- Apply vitamin A acid to thoroughly dry skin. Wet skin enhances penetration of the preparation, increasing the potential for irritation.
- Apply daily or as tolerated, e.g. alternate nights or less frequently, if necessary.

Advice to patient
Symptoms may become worse during the first few weeks of treatment because of the action of the medication on previously unseen comedones.
Improvement may take 4–8 weeks.
Erythema and peeling may occur.
During the early weeks, care should be taken about exposure to sunlight (including sun-lamps), as the antikeratinizing effect of topical vitamin A acid makes the skin more sensitive to sunburn.
Read the product information brochure.
Keep hands away from face.
Do not squeeze pimples or blackheads. Squeezing the skin may push the blackheads down into the skin, causing the follicles to rupture and making the acne worse.
Eat a healthy balanced diet: include fresh vegetables and reduce fatty and processed foods.
Wash face gently 3 times daily with mild soap and water to remove surface oil. Avoid irritants such as strong soaps.
Shampoo hair nightly or twice weekly with medicated shampoo. Keep hair off the face.
If the back is affected, use a bath brush when washing it.

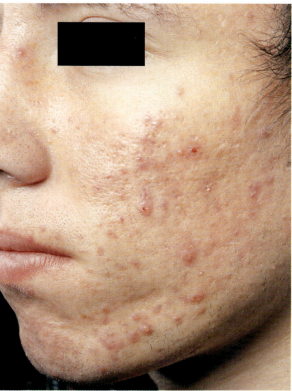

122

33   Injection of intra-lesional corticosteroids

Uses
To help to reduce inflammation in lesions, e.g. keloid scars (Figure **123**), lichen planus and acne cysts.
To try to stimulate re-growth of hair in alopecia areata (Figure **124**).

Equipment
Tray containing:
Prescribed medication for injection.
Sterile syringe and needles *or* needle-less pressure injector.
Alcohol-impregnated swabs.
Latex gloves.

Procedure
- Explain procedure to the patient and reassure throughout.
- Position patient comfortably and expose the area to be treated.
- Clean the area with an alcohol-impregnated swab.
- Inject the steroid into the lesion (Figure **125**).
- In alopecia areata, inject the steroid first evenly around the perimeter of the scalp area to be treated and then across the centre. This distributes the medication evenly across the lesion (Figures **126, 127**).
- Swab the area clean.
- Apply an adhesive plaster to trunk or limbs if necessary.

Advice to patient
The procedure may be repeated at intervals over a 3-month period.
Remove plaster when oozing has stopped.
Maintain usual skin care.
There may be no obvious response for 2–3 months in alopecia areata; in some cases the treatment is ineffective.

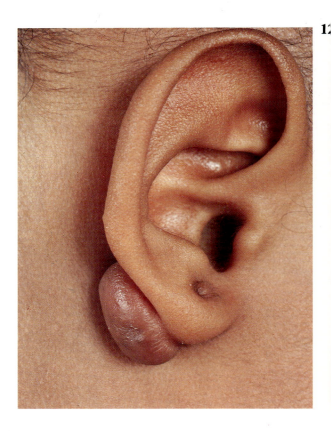

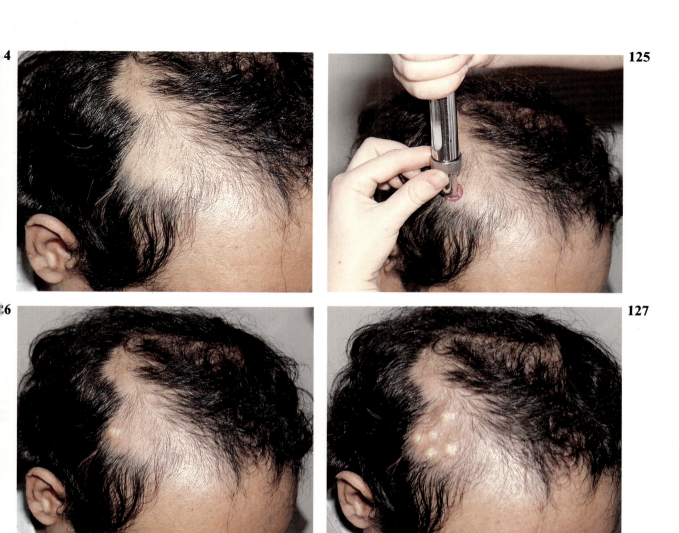

34   PUVA therapy (photochemotherapy)

This combines taking the drug methoxypsoralen with exposure of the skin to long-wave (320–400nm) ultra-violet light (UVA).

Use

To treat psoriasis (Figure **128**), eczema, polymorphic light eruption, vitiligo and mycosis fungoides.

Equipment

Methoxypsoralen as prescribed.
Protective spectacles for outdoors (for patient's on oral methoxypsoralen).
Protective goggles for use during UVA exposure.
UVA unit.

Procedure

Schedule for PUVA treatment

- Prior to starting therapy, the doctor explains the treatment, its benefits and possible side effects to the patient.
- The nurse explains the procedure in detail, measures the patient and checks the skin type carefully (Figure **129**), so that the dose of irradiation can be assessed and burning during treatment avoided.
- Methoxypsoralen tablets in the prescribed dose are given 2 hours before UVA exposure. Lotion is applied 15–20 minutes beforehand.

- Wearing the protective goggles, the patient is exposed to the prescribed dose of UVA (Figure **130**). For full body treatment the patient stands in a specially designed cabinet (Figure **131**). For small areas, e.g. palms, soles, a small UVA unit (Figures **132, 133**) may be used.
- In order to reassure the patient while enclosed in the cabinet, the nurse should maintain verbal contact.
- The individual dose and cumulative total of UVA is recorded after each treatment.
- The nurse checks the patient's skin before and after each treatment and reports any changes to the doctor.

Advice to patient

Protect skin from sunlight for 12 hours after taking the tablets.
Always wear protective spectacles (Figure **134**) for 12 hours after taking the tablets, as methoxypsoralens sensitises the eyes to light.
Avoid any other sunbathing or sunbeds while undergoing treatment.
Avoid perfumes, aftershaves, cosmetics or other scented toiletries as these may make the skin more sensitive to ultra-violet light.

128

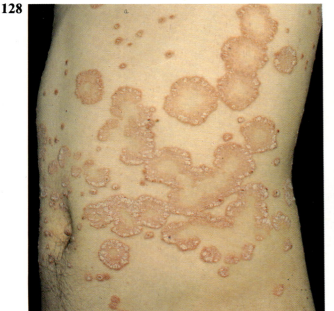

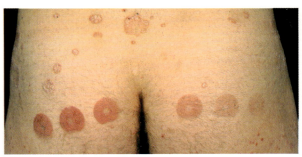

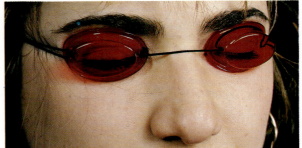

Inform the doctor or nurse of any other side effects, e.g. pricking or itching skin or nausea. Apply sufficient emollient after treatment to prevent skin from becoming too dry. Continue other topical treatments as prescribed. Photo-sensitive patients may need to fit ultra-violet light (UVL) filter blinds to windows.

N.B. Pathological skin changes may occur during the course of treatment.
Existing conditions which preclude treatment:
pregnancy, liver failure, renal failure, cardiac conditions, any previous treatments with arsenic (including arsenic-based cough medicines), psychological disturbance.

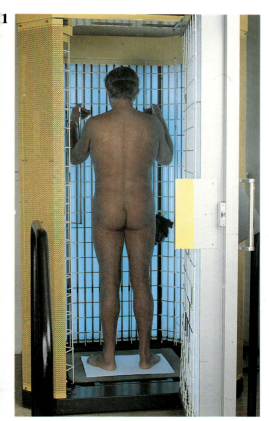

131

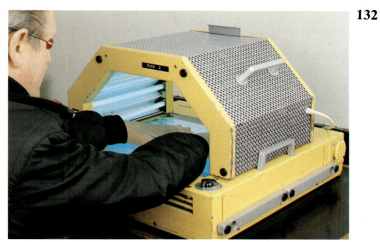

132

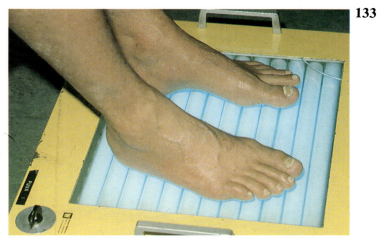

133

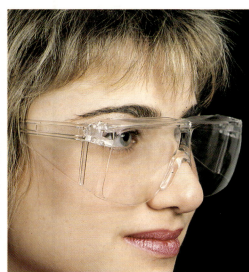

134

35   Acarus search

Use
To confirm a diagnosis of scabies infestation.

Equipment
Sterile Hagedorn needle or large sterile sewing needle.
Glass slide and cover slip.
5 per cent potassium hydroxide solution.
Microscope.

Procedure
- Explain procedure and reassure the patient.
- Position patient comfortably.
- Examine the patient for any sign of burrows. The common sites include finger webs, elbows, ankles and wrists (Figure **135**).
- Open the skin of the burrow until it is completely exposed.
- Remove debris from the burrow on the end of a needle (Figure **136**) and place on a glass slide with solution and cover slip.
- Examine specimen under microscope for presence of acarus (Figure **137**).
- Consult doctor for treatment.

135
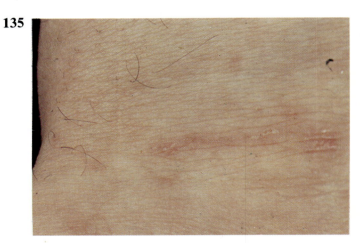

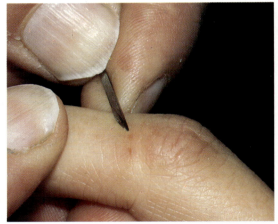

137
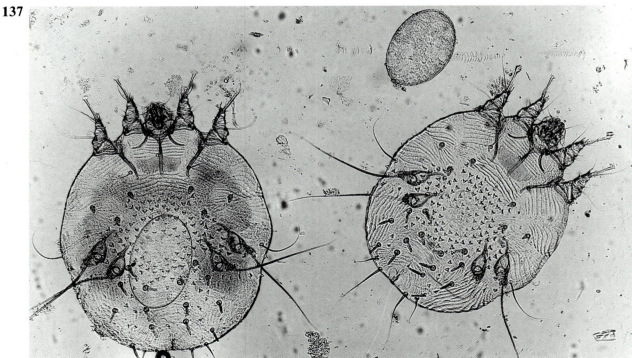

36 Treatment of infestation—scabies

Equipment
Prescribed scabicide (e.g. gamma benzene hexachloride for adults; malathion 0.5% for children; monosulfiram 25% for babies).
Cotton wool.
Small soft brush.
Bland ointment.

Procedure
- Take a soapy bath or shower to remove scaling from the crusts (Figures **138, 139**). Dry skin thoroughly. Allow to cool if gamma benzene hexachloride is being used, as flushed skin increases toxic hazard of the preparation and decreases its efficacy by conveying it away from the mites.
- Apply the scabicide as prescribed; it is usually more convenient to do so at bedtime.
- Apply lotion all over the body, except head and face, with cotton wool.

- Apply lotion carefully with the brush between fingers and toes and to soles of the feet (Figure **140**).
- Allow to dry.
- If prescribed, repeat the application next morning. Do not bath.
- After the prescribed length of time (8–24 hours) remove the lotion by bathing.
- Apply a bland ointment to the skin after completing treatment.

N.B. When it is necessary to wash the hands during treatment time, they should be re-treated immediately.

Advice to patient
Treatment should be repeated only on the doctor's instructions and not within 3 weeks. For maintenance of hygiene, it is advisable to put on freshly laundered or dry-cleaned clothes and change and wash all under-clothes, night-clothes and bed linen.
To eliminate mites, all the family members and close contacts must be treated simultaneously, whether or not they are infected. Symptoms do not usually occur until about 4 weeks following infestation.
Itching and irritation of the skin, caused by the treatment solution, may persist for some time and may be relieved by applying calamine cream. Any oral therapy prescribed for secondary infestation should be continued while carrying out topical treatment for scabies.

N.B. Monosulfiram is the preferred treatment for babies; other preparations should be avoided because of their side effects.

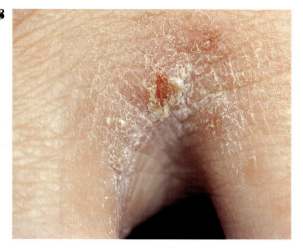

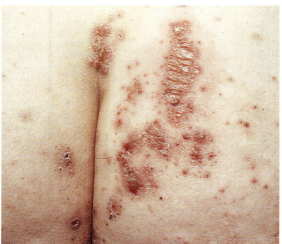

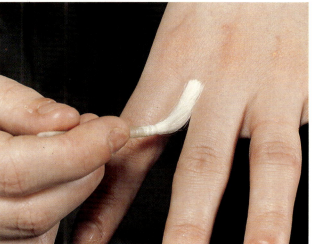

140

37 Treatment of infestation—head lice (pediculosis capitis)

Equipment
Fine-toothed nit comb.
Prescribed lotion (e.g. malathion 0.5%; carbaryl 0.5%), *or* prescribed shampoo.
Plastic cape.
Towel.
Shampoo.

N.B. Lotion is more effective than shampoo and helps to delay the emergence of resistant strains of lice.

Procedure
- Explain procedure to the patient.
- Seat the patient comfortably.
- Place cape around the patient's shoulders to protect clothing.
- *Using lotion:*
  (a) Apply lotion to the head (Figure **141**) and comb through the hair. Leave for the prescribed time.
  (b) Wash the head with an ordinary bland shampoo.

N.B. If parent or patient insists upon using a medicated shampoo, they must use a malathion shampoo after a malathion lotion and a carbaryl shampoo after a carbaryl lotion.

Using shampoo:
(a) Wet the head with warm water.
(b) Massage approx. 10ml of shampoo into wet head; leave for a minimum of 4 minutes.
(c) Rinse the head thoroughly with warm tap water to remove the shampoo.
(d) Allow hair to dry naturally (without using hair dryer).
(e) Repeat treatment twice with 3-day intervals between applications. This is to ensure that all louse eggs are dead and reduce the risk of resistant strains developing.
(f) Comb the hair with a nit comb between treatments until all lice are removed (Figure **142**).

Advice to patient
Use *either* a carbaryl *or* a malathion preparation but never both, to reduce the risk of resistant strains developing.
Children should be kept away from school until treatment is completed. School authorities should be notified and any other infested children treated.
Any secondary infection may require a suitable antibiotic.
Towels, combs, etc. must be kept separate.

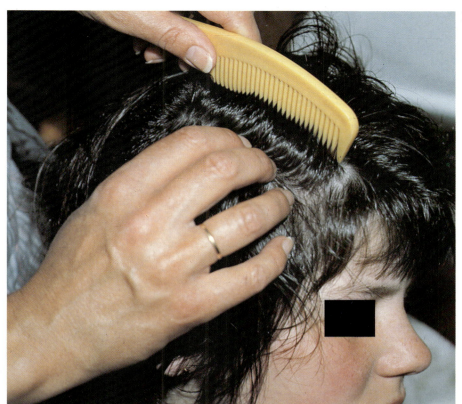

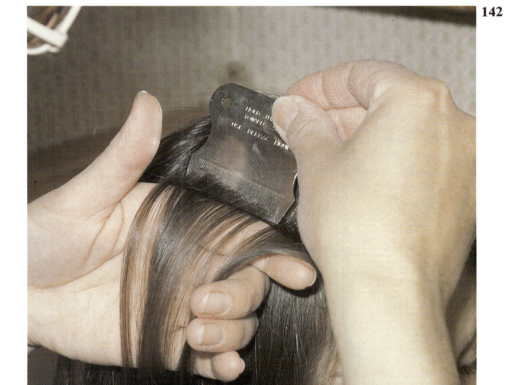

38   Dressings for ulcers and ulcerated skin

Dressing performance requirements contributing to the healing process were identified by Turner (1979):

1   Absorb exudate and toxic substances.
2   Maintain high humidity at the would/dressing interface.
3   Allow gaseous exchange and maintain pH.
4   Demonstrate impermeability to micro-organisms.
5   Insulate the wound from low temperature effects.
6   Ensure freedom from particles or other contaminants.
7   Allow removal without trauma at dressing change.

The development of new dressing products in the past decade has made it much easier to care for ulcerated skin and choose dressings based upon the Turner criteria.

Each patient must be assessed carefully so that the chosen dressing is appropriate for his/her individual needs. Non-adherent dressings are recommended for ulcerated conditions. When required, tubular or soft cotton bandages should be used to fix dressings in place. Adhesive tapes should be avoided for holding dressings in place on fragile skin. (See Procedure 16).

Non-adherent dressings

Type	Advantages	Disadvantages	Use
1 Tulle Gras	Maintains moist environment. Holds skin flat. May be vehicle for dispersal of anti-bacterials.	Requires absorbent pad to cover, and bandage to hold in place. Adheres to wound if allowed to dry out. Must be used in conjunction with other dressings.	Provides non-adherent base for an absorbent dressing. Skin grafts, superficial ulcers. Lubricates and protects fragile skin surfaces.
2 Films	Occlusive. Wound visible through dressing facilitates observation. Excess exudate can be aspirated using a syringe and needle without distributing dressing. Do not require changing daily.	Do not absorb exudate.	Stage I pressure sores, burns, intravenous cannula sites, donor sites.
3 Foams			
Sheets	Absorb exudate. Good insulators.	May be difficult to keep in place when large areas are involved.	Blistering disorders (Figure 36), (e.g. epidermolysis bullosa, pustular psoriasis, pemphigus), burns, erythroderma, leg ulcers.
Packs	Made in situ—ideal for cavity wounds. Absorb exudate. Good insulator. May be washed and replaced. Easy for patient's own use.	Rapidly granulating wounds require new dressings to be cast more frequently.	Cavity wounds, ulceration in mycosis fungoides, T-cell lymphoma.
4 Hydrogels	High water content. Absorb exudate. Easy to pour into difficult cavities or sinuses. Easily removed by irrigation.	Must be kept moist. Sheet form may damage healing skin if allowed to dry out. Requires dressing pad to cover and bandages to hold in place.	Burns, epidermolysis bullosa, ulcers, cavities.
5 Hydrocolloids	Occlusive. Absorb exudate. Good insulator. Patient can wash or bathe without disturbing underlying wound. Easily applied and removed. May be left in situ for up to one week. Patient can change own dressing.	Leaking from beneath dressing occurs in highly exudative wounds. Should not be used with severely infected wounds. May produce an unpleasant odour when leaking occurs or on changing.	Leg ulcers (Figures 143-146), pressure sores, burns, donor sites, ulcers in: pyoderma, gangrenosum, livedo reticularis, poikiloderma, mycosis fungoides.
6 Alginates Absorb exudate.	Biodegradable. Haemostatic. Require dressing pad to cover and Resultant gel easily flushed away. Useful in packing difficult cavities or sinuses.	Unsuitable in non-exudative wounds. epidermolysis bullosa, basal cell bandage to hold in place.	Highly exudative wounds; diabetic ulcers; donor sites; ulcers in: epithelioma, squamous cell epithelioma, pyoderma gangrenosum; packing for sinuses in difficult sites.

Vascular leg ulcers

When non-adherent dressings are used for ulcers related to an underlying vascular disroder, they must be combined with the appropriate degree of support, e.g. elastic support stockings, shaped-support tubular bandage or firm support bandaging. Patients with venous ulcers must be informed about the importance of exercise and the action of the 'calf-muscle pump'.

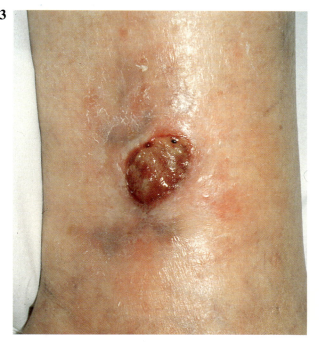

143

Ulcer on leg.

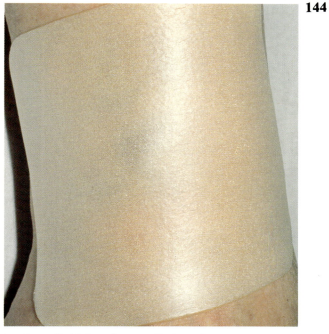

144

Hydrocolloid dressing applied to ulcer.

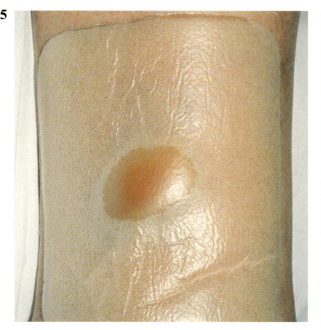

145

Hydrocolloid dressing after one week *in situ*.

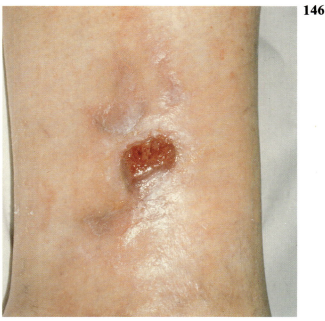

146

Ulcer after eight weeks' treatment with hydrocolloid dressing.

39 Hand care in dermatitis

Use
To speed healing and prevent a relapse
(Figure **147**).

(a) Hand washing
- Use lukewarm water and a mild soap without perfume, tar or sulphur.
- Use soap sparingly; rinse hands thoroughly.
- Dry carefully with a clean towel, especially between the fingers.
- Emulsifying ointment may be used instead of soap (see Figure **93**).

(b) Rings
- Avoid wearing rings.
- Clean rings frequently on the inside with a brush.
- Never wash the hands with soap when wearing a ring.

(c)
- Use running water for washing-up.
- Measure quantity of washing powder or detergent (powder or liquid) according to manufacturer's directions; otherwise the solution may be too strong.
- Keep packages clean to avoid irritation from detergent on the outside of the packet.

(d)
- Avoid direct contact with shampoo; use plastic gloves.
- Do not apply hair solution, hair cream or hair dye with ungloved hands.

(e) Avoid:
- Direct contact with metal, wax, shoe, floor, car, furniture or window polishes; detergents and other strong cleansing agents.
- Splashing solvents or stain-removers, e.g. white spirit, petrol, trichloroethylene, turpentine or thinners, on the skin.
- Peeling or squeezing citrus fruits with bare hands.

147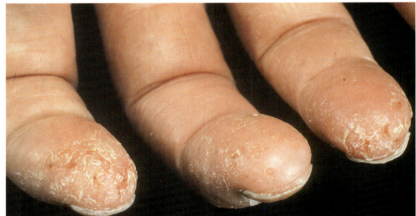

(f)
- Gloves for washing dishes or clothes (Figure **148**) should be plastic; rubber often causes dermatitis.
- Gloves should not be worn for more than 15–20 minutes at a time.
- Remove immediately if water enters a glove.
- Turn the gloves inside out and rinse under a hot water tap several times a week.
- Sprinkle gloves with unperfumed talc before using again to ensure that they are completely dry.

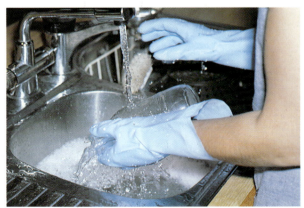

14

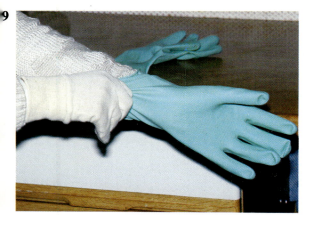

- Cotton gloves may be worn under plastic ones (Figure **149**) and should be washed frequently.
- It is recommended that people with hand dermatitis should use washing machines and dishwashers.

(g) Wear gloves in cold weather.

40　Advice for home treatment

- Plan treatment to fit a socially convenient time in the day/week.
- Try to maintain a regular pattern.
- When medicated or emollient baths are necessary, use a disposable plastic bath liner (see Figure **11**) to prevent staining of the bath. Care should be taken with children to avoid the risk of suffocation.
- Keep a set of cotton pyjamas/track suit/robe specifically for treatment times.
- Nylon stockings or a leotard help to keep ointments and creams in place.
- Shower caps or scarves may be used to cover head during scalp treatments.

- Keep emollient/moisturiser beside each basin; apply after every hand washing.
- Wrap up in a large bath sheet or towelling robe after emollient baths to absorb excess water droplets on skin.
  Do not rub skin dry—this would rub off the emollient.
- A medication applicator may be used to apply prescribed medication to inaccessible areas.
- Music at largo tempo (40–60 beats per minute) may calm children at bedtime (e.g. the slow movement of *Four Seasons* by Vivaldi).

41 Skin scrapings for mycological investigation

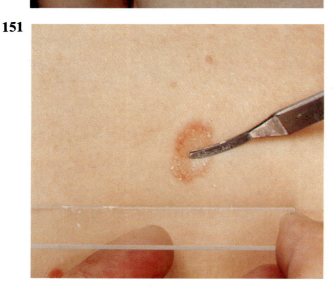

Use
To help diagnosis of fungal infections of the skin, (e.g. tinea corporis Figure **150**).

Equipment
   Blunt scalpel.
   Glass slide.
   Culture medium.
   Black paper.

Procedure
* Explain procedure to the patient.
* Position patient comfortably.
* Scrapings should be taken from the *periphery* of an active lesion. In vesicular eruptions a blister roof should be taken for examination.
* Using a blunt scalpel, scrape the skin scales on to a glass slide (Figure **151**) for direct examination under a microscope, and on to the culture medium for further identification of the organism. Scrapings may be wrapped in black paper before sending to the laboratory (Figure **152**).
* Apply a dressing to the lesion, if required.

Advice to patient
Consult the doctor for result of test and apply treatment as prescribed.

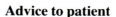

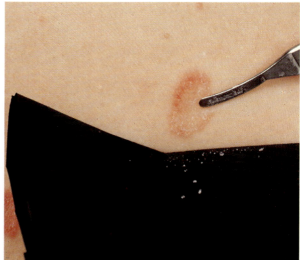

42 Curettage and cautery

Use
To remove superficial lesions, e.g. seborrhoeic warts.

Equipment
Sterile curettage set, comprising:
    Non-toothed forceps.
    Scissors.
    Curette or Volkmann's spoon.
    Gallipot.
    Gauze squares.
    Cotton wool balls.
    Tray.
Local anaesthetic materials, comprising:
    Syringe
    Needle, 23 gauge.
    Ampoule of local anaesthetic as
    prescribed.
Skin cleansing solution.
Surgeon's gloves.
Electro-cautery unit or silver nitrate stick.
Wound dressing.

Procedure
N.B. Aseptic technique must be used.
- The doctor explains procedure to the patient and obtains his/her consent. Reassure patient throughout.
- Position the patient lying down comfortably and expose the area to be treated (Figure **153**).
- The doctor prepares the sterile field, draws up and checks the local anaesthetic, swabs the area and injects the local anaesthetic.
- The doctor removes the lesion with the curette (Figure **154**); the nurse swabs away any blood with gauze.
- The doctor applies electro-cautery or the silver nitrate stick to the open wound area (Figure **155**).
- If possible, and providing it is acceptable to the patient, the wound should be left exposed. Wound dressing may be applied if required.

Advice to patient
A scab will form and should be left to separate spontaneously.
Keep scab clean and dry. If it becomes wet, gently pat dry with a clean paper tissue. Do not rub.
If the site becomes red or painful or leaks pus, consult the doctor.
After healing, a shallow pale depression will be left on the skin. This will fill out gradually with a good cosmetic result. Do not scratch off the scab as this may leave a more obvious scar.

3

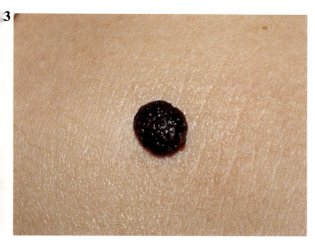

4

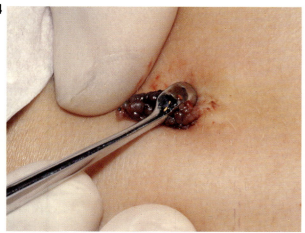

155

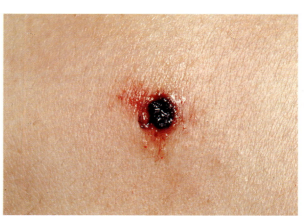

43   Skin biopsy

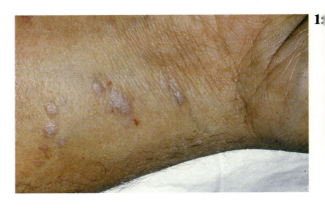

Use
To aid in diagnosis. (A specimen of skin, either
an ellipse or punch biopsy is excised for
histopathological examination.) This procedure is
usually performed under a local anaesthetic.

Equipment
Sterile biopsy/suture set, comprising:
    Scalpel handle.
    Toothed forceps.
    Non-toothed forceps.
    Spencer-Wells forceps.
    Needle holder.
    Scissors.
    Gallipot.
    Gauze squares.
    Cotton wool balls.
    Paper towels.
    Tray.
Local anaesthetic materials, comprising:
    Syringe
    Needle, 23 gauge.
    Ampoule of local anaesthetic as
    prescribed.
Scalpel blade.
Biopsy punch, if required.
Skin suture material.
Skin cleansing solution.
Surgeon's gloves.
Filter or blotting paper.
Specimen container.
Laboratory request form.
Adhesive wound dressing.

Procedure
N.B. Aseptic technique must be used.
- The doctor explains procedure to the patient
  and obtains his/her consent. Reassure patient
  throughout.
- Position the patient lying down comfortably
  and expose the area to be biopsied
  (Figure **156**).
- The doctor prepares the sterile field, draws up
  and checks the local anaesthetic, swabs the
  area and injects the local anasthetic,
  infiltrating the whole biopsy site.
- The doctor excises the skin in an ellipse
  (Figures **157 to 159**) or by using a biopsy punch
  (Figures **160 to 162**).
- The skin specimen is placed on the blotting
  paper. The nurse puts this in to the labelled
  specimen container.

- The doctor sutures the wound; the nurse swabs
  away any blood with gauze. A punch biopsy
  site may require only a skin-closure strip or
  cautery to control bleeding.
- Cut sutures about 0.5cm from the knot unless
  otherwise asked.
- Apply appropriate dressing. When possible
  patients with face, neck or scalp wounds should
  be encouraged to accept a plastic spray
  dressing, if they are not sensitive to it.

Advice to patient
Keep dressing clean and dry.
If the biopsy site becomes red or painful or leaks
pus, consult the doctor.
Attend for suture removal as instructed by the
doctor.
Do not apply topical steroids near the wound.

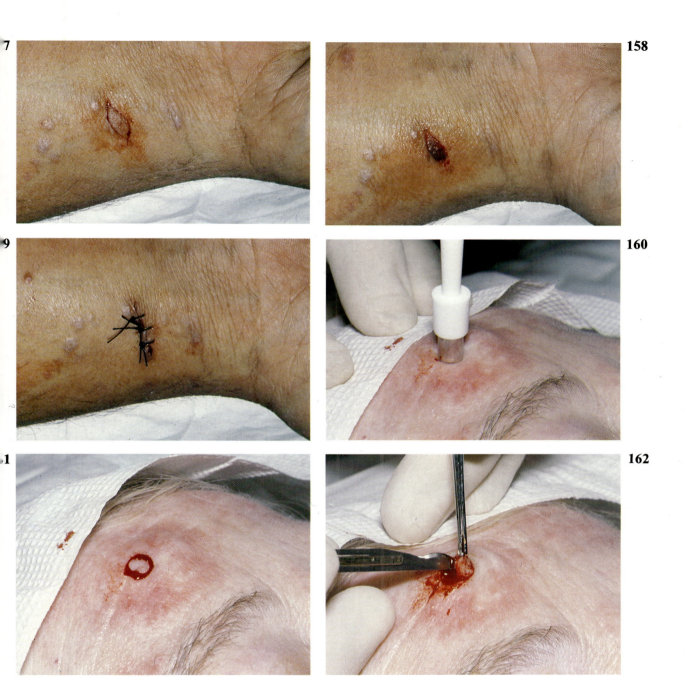

44   Patch testing

Use

To establish the diagnosis of contact dermatitis.

Equipment

Allergens to be tested.
Finn chambers (hypoallergenic tape, with aluminium chambers in strips of 10).
Filter-paper discs, to fit the chambers.
Pipette or orange sticks.
Skin-marking pen.
Scissors.
Hypoallergenic tape, 1cm width.
Reading template.
Solvent ether.
Gauze squares.

Procedure

Before the test

- The doctor takes a detailed history from the patient and decides upon the allergens to be tested.
- Warn the patient that two further visits at 48-hour intervals will be required to complete the test.
- The nurse prepares the prescribed allergens.
  - (a) Allergens diluted in petrolatum are applied in a line across the diameter of the chamber (Figure **163, 164**). When the tests are in place, the allergen spreads to fill the chamber but is contained within it.
  - (b) Allergens in solution form are applied using a pipette or orange stick to the filter disc, which is placed within the chamber. The filter disc should be completely moistened but not too saturated as to be unable to absorb all of the solution.

163
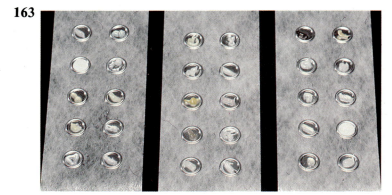

1
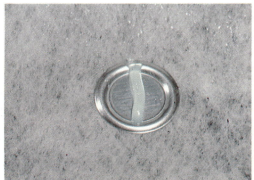

Application of the test

- Explain procedure to the patient before commencing and as it progresses.
- Sit the patient comfortably on a stool.
- Expose the patient's back. The upper back is the site normally used as it is a large, relatively flat area which is subject to pressure when the patient is lying down. If the back is unsuitable, e.g. if an acute eczematous reaction is present, alternative sites include abdomen, outer aspects of thighs and upper arms.
- No special skin preparation is required, apart from shaving the site in particularly hirsute patients.
- Fix the strip of chambers, starting at the bottom end of the tape to avoid dislodging any filter discs (Figure **165**).
- Ensure that the tape is properly fixed.
- Press firmly on each chamber to expel air and spread the allergen evenly over the area occluded by the chamber (Figure **166**).
- If several strips of chambers are used, fixed them in line where possible.
- Draw a pen mark on the patient's skin above and below the strip and number each column in order, to correspond with the allergens prescribed (Figure **167**).
- Record the allergen order on the diagram which the doctor refers to when reading the results (see page 70).

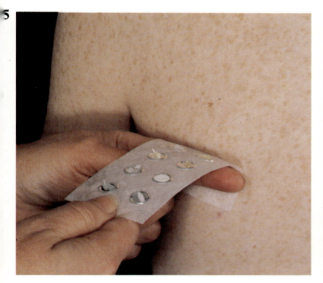

165

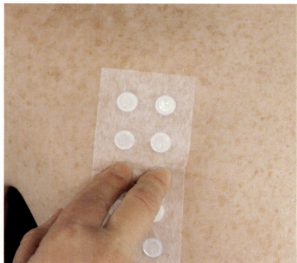

166

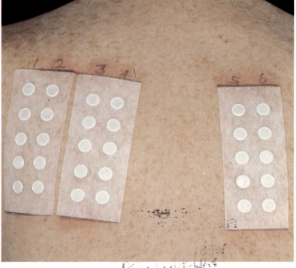

167

- Cover the numbers marked on the skin with 1cm hypoallergenic tape.
- Mark the numbers again on to the tape (Figure **168**). These marker tapes stay in place until the end of the test and are a guide for the doctor reading the results.

Advice to patient during the test
Test strips must stay in place for 48 hours, until the next visit, but remove the strip where any violent reaction occurs.
Keep test area dry.
Avoid extremely energetic activity which may dislodge strips or cause excessive sweating, e.g. squash, football.
Do *not* replace chambers which are exposed. It is impossible to replace them precisely and may confuse results.
Ensure that the 'marker tapes' stay in position.

Reading the test
On the patient's second visit:
- Check 'marker tape' and ensure that it is secure.
- Remove strips of tests.
- Check that a ring-shaped depression is visible (Figure **169**); this indicates that the tests have adhered successfully.
- Wipe the area with solvent ether to remove any remaining allergen or plaster marks.
- Allow 20–30 minutes for any plaster reaction to subside.

- The doctor uses the reading template to interpret the results (Figure **170**) and then records them.
- Further tests may be ordered to clarify a result, e.g. perfume ingredients where there is a positive reaction to the perfume-mix allergen. These are applied as above.
- Advise patient as before, emphasising the importance of keeping 'marker tapes' in position.
- Violent reactions to any allergens are usually treated locally, with a preparation such as a full strength topical corticosteroid ointment on a dry gauze dressing.

On the patient's third visit:
- Follow the same procedure as in 1–6 for the second visit.
- When reading and recording the results is completed (see page 70), remove all marker tapes and clean the patient's back.

Advice to patient
Avoid as much as possible any substance containing allergens to which you are sensitive. Take note of any substances containing the relevant allergen.
Consult a dermatologist, general practitioner or occupational health physician where appropriate, for further advice about treatment.

168

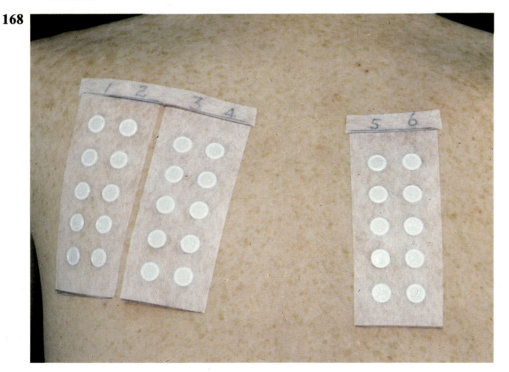

169

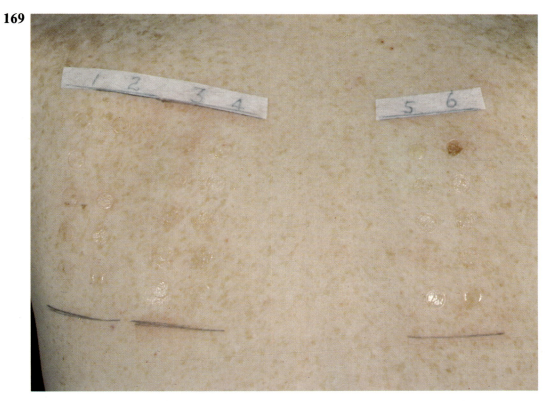

170

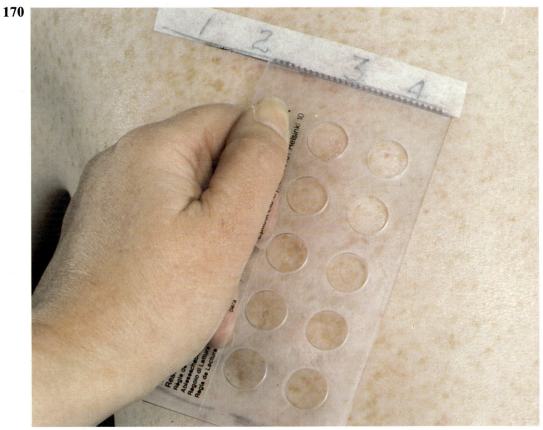

ATTACH
◄ LABEL
HERE
PLEASE

FEMALE

PATCH TESTS

NAME *BLOGGS, FREDA*

AGE 2 1

DATE 3 0 0 3 8 9

NUMBER A 1 2 3 4 5 6 X   PREVIOUS PATCH TEST

2 REFERRED BY

0 1 OCCUPATION

OWN ITEMS TO FOLLOW?

L.   R.

DIAGNOSIS CODE ☐☐ ☐ ☐☐ ☐☐ ☐

1 2 3 4   5 6
1 6 11 16   21 26
↓ ↓ ↓ ↓   ↓ ↓
5 10 15 20 25 27

TEST SUBSTANCES		2 days	4 days			2 days	4 days
1. Nickel Sulphate	5%			41.			
2. Bronopol				42.			
3. Colophony	20%			43.			
4. Chlorocresol	2%			44.			
5. P.P.D.	0.5%			45.			
6. M.B.T.	2%			46.			
7. Formalin	1%			47.			
8. Potassium Dichromate	0.5%			48.			
9. Wool Alcohols	30%			49.			
10. Epoxy Resins (Araldite)	1%			50.			
11. Primin	0.01%			51.			
12. Neomycin	20%			52.			
13. Cobalt Chloride	1%			53.			
14. Dowicil 200	1%			54.			
15. Parabens	15%			55.			
16. Thiuram-Mix	1%			56.			
17. Mercapto-mix	2%			57.			
18. Perfume-mix	8%			58.			
19. Black Rubber mix	0.6%			59.			
20. Sesquiterpene Lactone	0.1%			60.			
21. Quinoline mix	6%			61.			
22. Ethylenediamine	1%			62.			
23. P.T.B.P. Resin	1%			63.			
24. Kathon CG	100ppm			64.			
25. Caine mix	25%			65.			
26. Balsam of Peru	25%			66.			
27. Imidazolidinyl Urea (G115)	2%			67.			
28. Tixocortol Pivolate	1%			68.			
29. Ceto-Stearyl Alcohol	20%			69.			
30.				70.			
31.				71.			
32.				72.			
33.				73.			
34.				74.			
35.				75.			
36.				76.			
37.				77.			
38.				78.			
39.				79.			
40.				80.			

Common dermatological disorders

The following illustrations show a selection of skin problems which the dermatological nurse will have to deal with. The appropriate treatments for these can be found in the atlas.

Eczematous eruptions

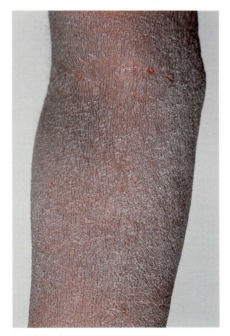

1   Atopic eczema

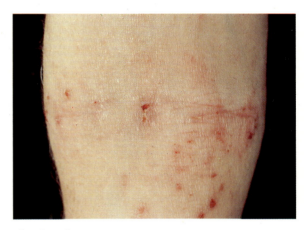

3   Contact dermatitis (nickel sensitivity)

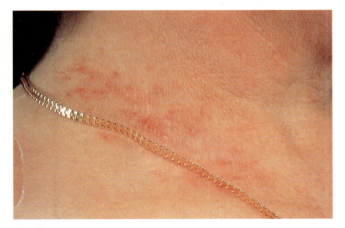

2   Atopic eczema

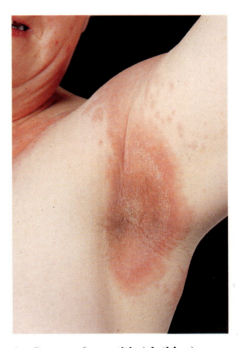

4   Contact dermatitis (clothing)

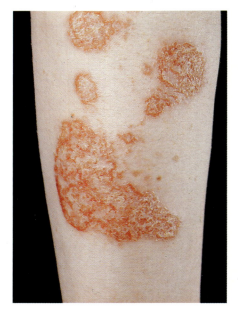

5   Discoid eczema

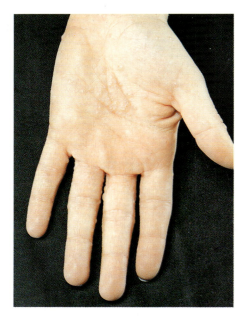

6   Vesicular hard eczema

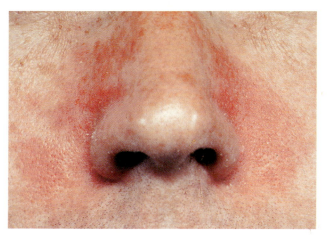

7   Seborrhoeic eczema

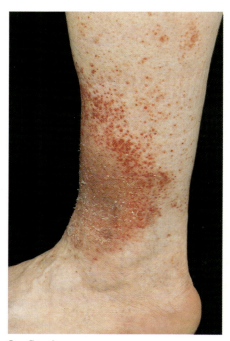

8   Stasis eczema

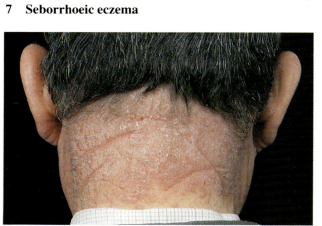

9   Photo-sensitivity

Psoriasis

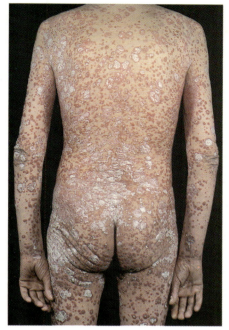

10   Generalised plaque psoriasis

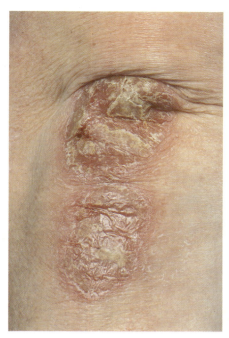

11   Psoriatic plaque

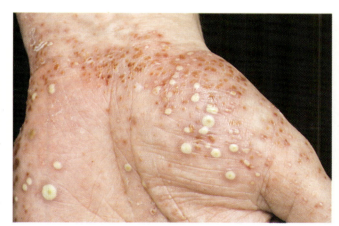

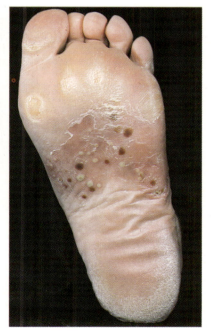

12a and 12b   Palmar/plantar pustulosis (pustular psoriasis of palms and soles).

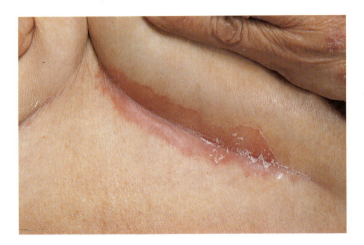

13 Flexural psoriasis

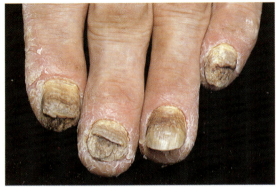

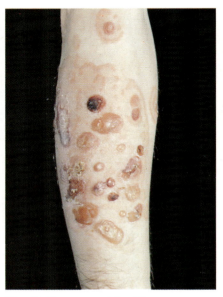

14 Generalised erythrodermic psoriasis

15 Nail psoriasis

Blistering disorders

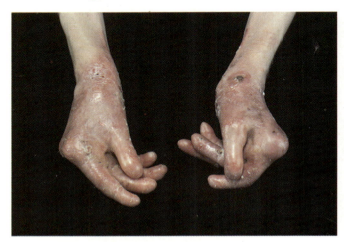

16 Dystrophic epidermolysis bullosa

17 Bullous pemphigoid

Skin infections

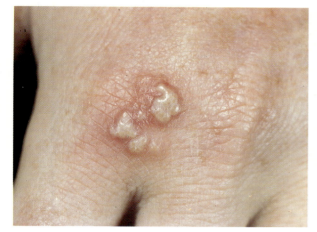

18   Herpes simplex

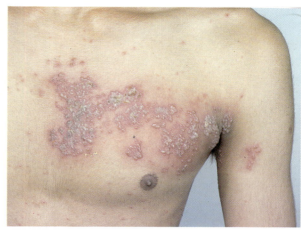

19   Herpes zoster

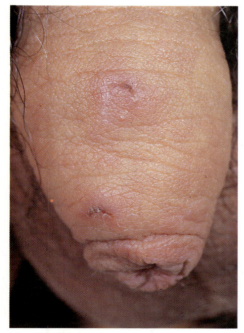

20   Scabies

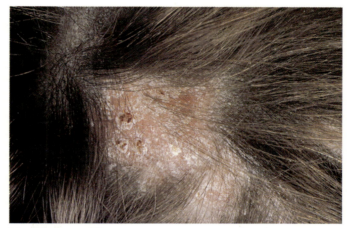

21   Tinea capitis

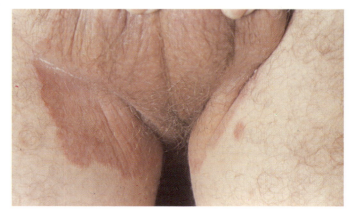

22   Tinea cruris

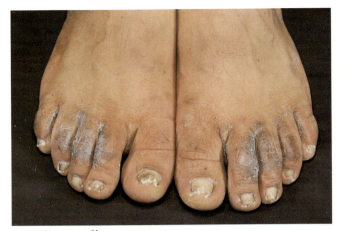

23 Tinea pedis

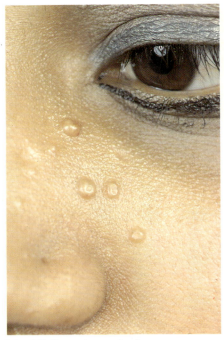

24 Molluscum contagiosum

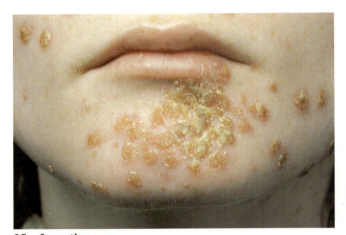

25 Impetigo

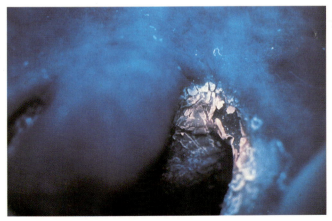

26 Erythrasma

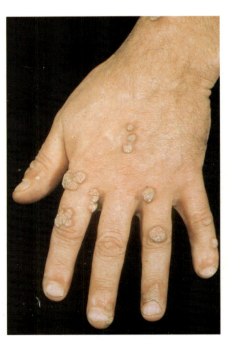

27 Warts (viral)

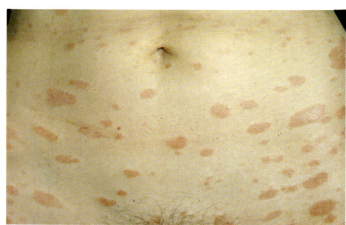

28 Pityriasis rosea

Tumours

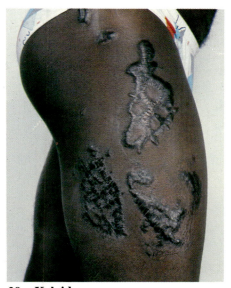

29 Keloid

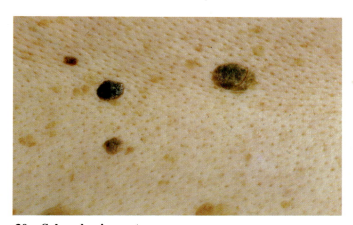

30 Seborrhoeic warts

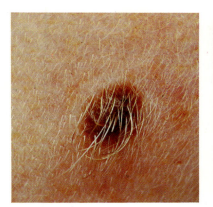

31 Pigmented naevus

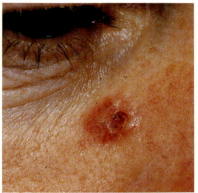

32 Basal cell epithelioma

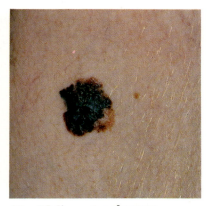

33 Malignant melanoma

Bibliography

Buxton, P K (1988), *ABC of Dermatology*, BMA, London

Cronin, E (1980) *Contact Dermatitis*, Churchill Livingstone, London

David, J A (1986) Wound Management, Martin Dunitz, London

Fincham-Gee, C & Stone, L A, Chapter Eds., (1988) Skin, *Nursing*, 3: 29

Fregert, S (1981) *Manual of Contact Dermatitis*, 2nd Edn., Munksgaard, Copenhagen

Fry, L, Wojnarowska, F & Shahrad P, (1981) Illustrated Encyclopedia of Dermatology, MTP Press Ltd, London

Hughes, G V R, *Lupus: a guide for Patients*, Rheumatology Department, St. Thomas' Hospital, London

Levene, G M & Calnan C D, (1974) A Colour Atlas of Dermatology, Wolfe Medical Publications, London

McKie, R, (1983) *Eczema and Dermatitis*, Martin Dunitz, London

Malten, K E, Nater, J P & Venketel, W G (1976) *Patch-Testing Guidelines*, Dekker & van de Vegt

Marks, R, (1984), *Acne*, Martin Dunitz, London

Marks, R, (1981) *Psoriasis*, Martin Dunitz, London

Maunder, J W (1981), Clinical and Laboratory Trials employing carbaryl against the Human head-louse, Pediculosis Human Capitis (de Gear), *Clinical and Experimental Dermatology*, 6, pp 605-612

Meneghini, C & Bonifazi E, ex. Marks, (1986), *An Atlas of Paediatric Dermatology*, Martin Dunitz, London

Murphy, G (1987) *Answers to Acne*, Optima (Macdonald & Co) London

Murray, D (1981) *The Anti-Acne Book*, Arlington Pocket Books, London

Orton, C (1981) *Learning to live with Skin Disorders*, Souvenir Press, London

Rook, A, Wilkinson, D S & Ebling A, (1979) *A Textbook of Dermatology*, 3rd edn., Blackwell Scientific, London

Runne, V & Kunze, J (1982), Short duration ('Minutes') therapy with dithranol for psoriasis: a new outpatient regimen, *British Journal of Dermatology*, 106, pp 135-139

Sidhanee, A C & Stone, L A, Chapter Eds., (1983) Skin, *Nursing*, 2: 9 and 10

Stone, L A (1989) Care of the Patient with a Skin Disorder or Burn, *Lippincott Medical-Surgical Nursing*, 2nd Edn., Chapter 11, Harper & Row, London

Tring, F C (1981) Warts and their treatment, *Nursing Times*, 77: pp 1415-1417

Turner, T D (1985) Semiocclusive & Occlusive Dressings: An environment for healing: the role of occlusion, *The Royal Society of Medicine*, International Congress and Symposium Series No. 88: pp 5-14

Further information may be obtained from the various local patient or self-help groups, e.g. The Psoriasis Association, DEBRA (Dystrophic Epidermolysis Bullosa Research Association).